THE OTHER SIDE
OF THE STORY _____

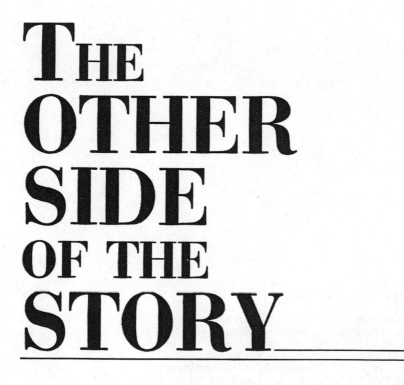

——JODY POWELL

THE
OTHER
SIDE
OF THE
STORY

William Morrow and Company, Inc. | New York | 1984

Library of Congress Catalog Card Number: 84-60200

ISBN: 0-688-03646-5

Printed in the United States of America

First Edition

1 2 3 4 5 6 7 8 9 10

BOOK DESIGN BY VICTORIA HARTMAN

This book is dedicated to the memory of my father, who I wish had been here to see it all, and to my mother, whose twenty-five years of teaching American history and government have undoubtedly contributed more to the strength of the Republic than most of the people, programs, and policies mentioned in this book.

Also to Nan and Emily. They know why.

ACKNOWLEDGMENTS _____

The journey from book proposal to completed manuscript, particularly for one's first book, is an intimidating and humbling experience. Second only to that is the task of acknowledging the debt owed to all those who made the trek possible.

The many journalists who contributed to this effort, through advice and criticism and, most important, information, must be thanked as an anonymous group. To link their names to a book that is likely to be less than well received by many of their colleagues would be the height of ingratitude.

The same can be said regarding former colleagues from the White House, whose assistance should not be repaid by drawing them into the line of fire.

There are some, however, who are already too closely identified with this work to escape, and they may be mentioned personally:

My longtime secretary, assistant, and straw boss, Carolyn Shields. Without her I would never have survived the White House or the writing of this book.

Esther Newberg was an ever-available source of advice and encouragement that went far beyond what anyone has a right to expect from an agent.

My editor, Bruce Lee, who got me on the right track and kept me there.

Ken Johnson, Jon Senderling, and the rest of the good people at the *Dallas Times Herald*, who graciously permitted the time off I so desperately needed when the going was the most frantic.

Finally, there is the gentleman from Plains who allowed me to be there and see it all (but who should not be held in any way accountable for the opinions and observations expressed in this book). His quiet determination to do what he saw as right despite the consequences is an example I shall never forget. I hope I will occasionally be able to live up to it. He deserved so much better than he got.

CONTENTS

INTRODUCTION _____

On January 20, 1981, when a new administration took over the White House, I had deep reservations about the way the fourth estate covers government, and the White House in particular. In some cases my reservations bordered on resentment. At that moment my wounds were deep and fresh, and it seemed to me that if I was going to write a book about the press I would have to design some structure or methodology that would restrain my tendency to let those wounds show.

The more I tried to play that game and write that book, however, the more frustrated and uneasy I became. "If you want to call someone an SOB," I had always been told, "do it to his face." I was doing just the opposite. As George Wallace used to say, I was "pussyfooting around."

Worse, I was using a dodge that always sent me up the wall when I saw or suspected its use by a reporter: the promulgation of subjective, value-laden personal opinion in the guise of something more objective and analytical.

The problem with that book was that it was not me. However, the time I spent interviewing reporters and editors for "that book" was not wasted, because it furnished the basis for what follows. More important, it convinced me that my original instincts when I left the White House were the right ones.

What follows, then, is not objective. It is how I felt, and still feel, and why I feel that way. It is my reaction to the reporting of news that I witnessed from the vantage point of four years in the White House Press Office.

In the three years since I left the White House I have been able to view it all from a more detached perspective. From that has come a better understanding of why things happened the way they did. But there has been no lessening in my belief that in too many cases what happened was wrong. I am still as upset, and in some cases even angry, about some of those experiences as I was at the time.

Where specific examples of what was said, done, and written are used, I have done my best to be accurate and complete. I have not knowingly concealed things that happened in the White House that might undermine my criticism of the way a story was handled.

When they were willing to cooperate, and most of them were, I have given the reporters who wrote or broadcast the story a chance to have their say, and I have tried to reflect their views accurately.

But this book is not objective in the sense of being balanced or fair. It does not reflect good, bad, and indifferent reporting in their real-life proportions. White House correspondents will look in vain for those scoops and pieces of insightful analysis that were right on the money—the ones that even I admitted were accurate, although painful. What they will find, for the most part, are the news stories that seemed to me, then and now, to be wrong, unsupportable, and unfair.

There is one area in which I have striven mightily to be fair and complete, and have undoubtedly fallen short. That is the assessment of my own mistakes. My reasons for even making the effort are twofold, and, I must admit, not altogether unselfish.

First, I have always been put off by Washington books of the "if they had only listened to me" variety. Such attempts to make oneself look good at the expense of friends and colleagues, or even the President who provided the opportunity to someday write such a book, seem to me to be one of the lower forms of human endeavor.

When Joe Califano produced the first such tome from the Carter administration, my generalized distaste became quite specific. I thought his criticisms of others might have been taken more seriously if he had been somewhat more willing to acknowledge that somewhere along the way he, Joe Califano, might have made a mistake, a misstep, or even a judgment that could be reasonably questioned with the benefit of hindsight.

And so I hope that throwing in a bit of self-deprecation now and then will lend more credibility to the criticisms I make of others.

Actually, I guess there is another reason for my attempting to write about my own shortcomings: that universal wish among writers that things will change because of what they write. I cannot honestly say that I expect to make straight the crooked way of American journalism, but I can at least hope to ease somewhat the tortured path of future press secretaries. Perhaps if I recount enough of my mistakes, one of my successors will say someday, "Well, I certainly won't be tempted to try such and such. Powell made that mistake back in '78 and damn near destroyed the President and the Republic."

Of course there are dangers in trying to have the thing both ways, to come across both as the avenging angel and as the nice, modest fellow who is quite willing to confess his own sins. One problem is that no matter what people say about understanding that everyone is human and therefore frail, they really do not like to believe that those who sit in judgment might be sinful themselves. This problem would bother me more if I thought there was any chance that the reader could be convinced that a press secretary was perfect, whatever I said.

The second danger is the flip side of the first: that in any given situation the reader will be inclined to excuse or mitigate the faults of journalists based on the realization that the press secretary could have handled the situation better. "After all," the reader may be tempted to say, "maybe those poor reporters wouldn't have made such a mess of it if Mr. Powell had known what he was doing."

In the face of such a discouraging possibility, I can only say, "Please, don't!" It will only confuse the issue. I promise not to use the shortcomings of journalists to excuse my stupidities if the reader will try to apply the same "No excuse, sir" standard to them.

In return, I will give fair warning about another thing this book is not. Those looking for a behind-the-scenes critique of the Carter administration, replete with backroom anecdotes about who took what position on this or that controversial decision and who was responsible for this or that mistake, will be disappointed.

It is not that I believe that President Carter or the administration he headed was perfect, nor were there no decisions that I thought then and think now were mistakes.

What I do think is that there are plenty of people who have written, and will write, about the mistakes and problems. Some of these people know what they are talking about. A lot do not. Furthermore, if I began listing those instances where I think the President would have been better off taking my advice, I would also have to deal with all those situations in which the country is a safer, better place to live in because he didn't—and I don't feel up to writing a book that long.

There is, in short, no danger that the shortcomings of the Carter administration, real or imagined, will be neglected. My purpose is to deal with the shortcomings of those who covered and critiqued the administration. That is unplowed ground.

At this point, readers who are particularly taken with one form of political ideology or another may be thinking that they are about to have their pet theory about the press confirmed: that the problem with American journalism is that all the reporters are snot-nosed, left-wing kids who never did a real day's work in their lives; or that the problem is self-satisfied, fat-cat editors and publishers who have no understanding of or feeling for the plight of the poor and downtrodden.

I must again give fair warning that these readers will be disappointed.

I would feel worse about their disappointment if I had a better opinion of ideology of any description, but I do not. It is the handmaiden to self-righteousness and abuse of power, the refuge of the slow mind and faint heart. It is responsible for as much error, waste, needless disputation, and downright foolishness as any other invention of the human mind. I am content to take religion on faith because there is no way to prove or disprove its basic assumptions, but not politics. We have been testing political ideologies since day one, and the only thing that proves out every time is that none of them work.

As I was saying, or was about to say, before that essential digression, the principal problem with journalism is not political or ideological bias. It exists, but it just does not count for much. And when it does count, it sometimes has unanticipated consequences, as we shall see.

In the first place, that is one disease that journalistic training seems to be successful in inoculating against. Reporters are taught to avoid partisanship and politics no matter what, that politics is a tacky business that decent folk don't bother with anyway; and if that's not enough, playing to a political preference is more likely to be spotted and punished than any other transgression.

Secondly, most journalists do not care that much about ideology. They are about as apolitical a group as you are likely to find anywhere. In that sense they make the supposedly apolitical military look like party hacks. They vote because that is what civic-minded Americans are supposed to do, and they are interested in politics because the job requires it. But when it comes down to this or that political theory or party, they mostly just do not care.

Columnists and commentators are, of course, a special case. But they are supposed to be writing opinion anyway, and political bias should not be a problem. It becomes one occasionally among columnists who report and investigate as well as pontificate. Some of these people have been known to make up, or willfully distort, information to support their political preferences.

However, that problem belongs in a more general category: the willingness to lie and deceive. It belongs there, because making things up and not telling the truths are means that journalists of various descriptions use to achieve a number of ends, the promotion of a political idea or party being one of the least common.

The major bias in journalism, it seems to me, the one most likely to promote deception and dishonesty, has its roots in economics. The fact is that news has to sell, or those who report it and edit it will find themselves searching for a new job. And that creates a bias to make news reports interesting.

There is nothing wrong with that on its face. The problems arise when the requirements of being interesting and being accurate part company. What constraints then operate to push the reporter or editor toward accuracy? There are some. My argument, however, is that they are and they will always be inadequate unless there are some changes in the way the news business operates.

It is not that every reporter writes every story with the next annual report of his news organization uppermost in his mind. In fact, most of them swear up and down that this is the furthest thing from the truth, and they are right. The bias is more subtle than that, but not particularly complicated. That *post hoc* rationale is usually expressed as "If it's not interesting enough to make people want to read or watch or listen, it's a wasted effort."

There is some truth to that contention, but it is a dangerous truth. It serves not to restrain but to promote self-interested behavior. It also reflects a measure of condescension toward the public that is not particularly attractive, which is yet another issue.

As might be expected, reporters who play the make-it-interesting game with the greatest zeal are often the ones who are most handsomely rewarded. Some who cover and comment upon the actions of senators, congressmen, Cabinet members, and the senior White House staff are paid considerably more than those they are paid to watch. (An interesting situation in which society pays more for the watchdog than for the house.)

Thus, members of the press wrestle with the most basic and pervasive of human motivations: greed and ambition. If you want to get ahead, it is good to be accurate, but you had damn well better be interesting and salable.

This ambition business can produce some strange behavior and occasional recriminations among journalists themselves. One of the more exciting afternoons around the White House Press Office was the day Lesley Stahl of CBS did a number on Judy Woodruff of NBC.

Judy was on the North Lawn of the White House, where the network correspondents do their stand-ups, with an exclusive on an upcoming Cabinet appointment. (Because of the close working conditions there—only one angle will give you just the right shot of the impressive, floodlit North Portico as a backdrop—correspondents are mostly on their honor not to steal stories.) In this case, Lesley's ambition got the better of her honor; hearing from her crew that Judy had something big, she slipped out to eavesdrop, then hurried back inside to do a radio spot that went on the air almost immediately, thus scooping Judy on her own story.

That produced major indignation among journalists of every description. Even Lesley's colleagues at CBS had little to say in her defense. Lesley, however, was not apologetic and has made clear that she might well do the same thing again under similar circumstances.

All of which is fine and interesting, particularly if you note that the universal condemnation of this crass yielding to temptation resulted from the fact that the victim was a fellow journalist. Those of us watching with some amusement from the sidelines had no doubt that if the wounded party had been one of us, the outrage among Lesley's colleagues would have been slim to nonexistent.

Unfortunately, the desire to be interesting has consequences that go beyond stealing another reporter's story. Objectivity, the eternal bugaboo of journalists that is certainly unattainable *in toto*, is also affected. No one can learn enough about a subject to discuss it intelligently without forming some opinions along the way. Those opinions inevitably color and shape perceptions of events that follow. Indeed, one can reasonably argue that total objectivity can only be the product of total indifference or of total ignorance.

The recognition that complete objectivity is not possible, nor even worthwhile at the price of ignorance and indifference, does not eliminate the problem. There are those, less common now than a few years back, who will argue that it does. They are the journalistic equivalent of those in politics who take the admonition that "ye have the poor always with you" as an excuse not to worry about starving children.

For journalists, the problem of identifying biases is complicated, or should be, by the fact that the sources of most stories are other subjective individuals. Those who read such a report have a right to know something about the possible prejudices of its sources. This is particularly true when the sources are not identified by name. Every "blind quote" cannot be accompanied by a three-thousand-word professional and personal profile, but, once again, the impossibility of achieving perfection does not eliminate the possibility of improvement.

If a reporter's source has a clear and identifiable stake in the outcome of the issue under discussion, the reader ought to be told, but usually is not. Comments from "informed sources" on the tar baby incident would be infinitely more informing to the reader if it were known whether they came from an associate of Brer Rabbit or Brer Fox.

To make matters worse, it is not unheard of for reporters to partially identify the source of a blind quote in a way that will give the quote a little extra zing and make the story more interesting and salable. The ideal is the "Even his wife thinks he's a jerk" quote. Thus, a verbal swipe at a President is better if it comes from a senator of his own party, and even better if it comes from an official of his own administration.

It may be, however, that the administration official is a member of the domestic policy staff commenting on a decision to increase the defense budget at the expense of domestic programs, and the Democratic senator may still be smarting from an unsuccessful race against the President a few years back. If the reporter knows these things, those who read the story and the quotes have a right to some inkling about them too. As we shall see in the chapter on Hamilton Jordan, that information is often concealed from the public, particularly if it might take the edge off the point the reporter is trying to make.

At its extreme, the problem of blind quotes goes all the way to the manufacturing of, or doctoring of, comments to give a story more punch. Few journalists deny that this takes place, although I could find none who would admit to doing it themselves. Few outsiders who have watched news reporting over any extended period of time doubt that anonymous quotes are occasionally cooked up or rewritten. But it is one of the most difficult offenses to prove since it involves the logical impossibility of proving a nonevent.

Occasionally, however, such behavior is observable. Early in the administration, *Newsweek* was looking for a sharp quote to support a story. In an interview with National Security Adviser Zbigniew Brzezinski they got something like what they wanted. *Newsweek* editors in New York rewrote his comments to conform more closely to the story line and to be more provocative, and sent them back to Brzezinski.

Would he be willing to approve this "revised" set of comments so they could be used in the magazine?

Brzezinski flatly refused. *Newsweek* could use what he said, as he said it, or nothing at all.

If the source had been a lower-level official, speaking anonymously instead of on the record, one cannot help but wonder whether any attempt would have been made to seek approval for the doctoring.

Several reporters at *Newsweek* were as appalled by the incident as those of us in the White House, although less inclined to view it as symptomatic of a general abuse of blind quotes in the news business.

The problems described in the last few pages are not terribly original or surprising. They are, in fact, all too familiar. The fact is that there are large and powerful groups throughout society whose internal goals and imperatives are in conflict with the public good and the general welfare. Even the rationalization process by which the pursuit of selfish goals is ascribed to unselfish motivations is not a new thing to most of us, primarily because we use it ourselves most days of the week.

Journalists share the problems and the rationalization with doctors, lawyers, farmers, business, labor, political parties, and much of organized religion. What sets journalists apart is that no one is looking over their shoulder, at least no one who is in a position to do much about what is seen.

It is not that editors do not edit or that all reporters are without scruples. Far from it. But any careful observer can quickly detect large differences in the amount of editorial scrutiny among news organizations and the fatal weakness is that almost all the checks and constraints are located *within the organization*. The only judge of the performance of the *Washington Post* is the *Washington Post*—or at least the only judge in a position to do much about it. The same is true for CBS News, *Time* magazine, and so on down the list.

The process is roughly equivalent to saying, "Well, I think the President and his chief of staff are decent fellows on the whole; let's forget about this investigative reporting business and trust them to make sure that the executive branch does its duty."

We leave the question of right and wrong in the press, unlike other powerful institutions in our society, to the individual consciences of reporters and editors.

I am a great believer in individual conscience. But one of the things I believe most strongly about it is that it usually is not adequate. I am enough of a Calvinist to think that the best way to get people to do what is right is to introduce into their hearts and minds a healthy fear of what will happen to them if they do wrong. The fear that mistakes, incompetence, or malice will be discovered and exposed and those responsible will suffer the consequences simply does not exist in journalism to the extent that it should; or even, I would argue, to the extent that it does in many other powerful institutions.

Of course, in addition to the requirement to be interesting journalists are prey to most of the other dangers that afflict the rest of us when we try to approach any subject objectively. Some of them are personal: friendship—and in some cases more intense relationships—plus antipathy, snobbery, and insecurity, to name just a few.

There are also pitfalls that combine personal professional considerations in a mix too complex to analyze: the extension of the legitimate need to protect sources to include the questionable and all too common practice of promoting and rewarding them, for example. It is generally understood by Washington insiders that one of the best ways to keep your name out of the news in an unflattering context is to be a ready source of information, preferably unflattering, about others. Like other creatures, reporters tend not to bite the hand that is feeding them.

Which reminds me that I should say something about reporters as individuals, though I am somewhat hesitant to do so for fear it may be taken as pandering or an attempt to sugarcoat what is to follow. The sordid truth is that I have actually become somewhat fond of the breed. Several have become friends; I trust they will remain so after this book is published. They are as interested and interesting a group of people as one would ever want to meet. Few people of moderate means get to go to as many interesting places and see as many thought-provoking things as do journalists. And few are as good at telling about it, which is not surprising, I guess, since that is the reason they went and saw in the first place.

Furthermore, and this may surprise some, most reporters have fewer and less serious ego problems than most other influential people. This is particularly true among print journalists, where there still lingers an ethos from an earlier day: the idea that reporters are not supposed to be personalities, that they should be a little frayed about the edges, just working stiffs trying to get at the truth.

That image is less apparent, although not altogether invisible, among columnists and television journalists. It is hard to be humble when you are invited to dine with Presidents and/or pull down several hundred thousand dollars a year. Even among most of the elite in the press, however, there is a willingness, at the personal level, to get in and mix it up, to argue, cuss, and discuss without taking offense.

I occasionally debated with Frank Moore, who was in charge of White House liaison with the Congress, in a not altogether serious fashion, about who had the worst job. He insisted that I did. I argued to the contrary. The major point in my case was not who caught the most hell, but who was in a better position to give a bit of it back. On that dimension I had an undisputable advantage.

I could, and often did, express my reservations about a story in the most blunt and colorful language I could command. If reporters, as they did on occasion, felt that I was behaving like a jackass, they said so. And I felt free to respond with the equivalent of "So's your mother."

For Frank to have dealt similarly with an irate and obnoxious member of Congress, of which there is always an ample supply, would have produced a political crisis. There would have been denunciations and resolutions on the floor of both houses, and the President would have been called upon to deliver Mr. Moore's head along with a personal apology.

I particularly recall, on that score, a return flight from Europe in 1979. The trip had been a backbreaker for the press and the White House staff, and everyone was glad to be headed home. The final leg of a foreign trip is always a gas on the press plane, and I usually found an excuse to be there instead of on Air Force One.

This particular flight was actually unremarkable until the last couple of hours. A crowd of us were singing a little country music and a sprinkling of hymns to the accompaniment of Bobby "Hoss" Law, a White House Transportation Office staffer who also picks a fine guitar, when up strolled Sam Donaldson. His purpose was to needle me about some unhappy incident on the trip, which he had already milked for all it was worth on *World News Tonight*. I was in no mood for such foolishness, being smack in the middle of trying to remember the third verse of "I'm So Lonesome I Could Cry," and I proceeded, with sure intent and malice aforethought, to empty a glass of wine on ABC's senior White House correspondent.

In addition to being decidedly impolite, it was an incredibly stupid thing to do. The mavens of Washington gossip were scouring the gutters for evidence that the Carter crowd ate with their fingers and did not wear socks. I had just given them enough to wallow in for a month.

The next morning I called Sam to apologize. He laughed it off, and that was the end of it. Not a word ever appeared in print anywhere. All it would have taken was one phone call to put me in serious trouble. In fact, all he had to do was tell the story around town, and someone else would surely have made the call; but he did not, and he never mentioned the incident again.

The difference between my clientele and Frank Moore's was that he could not even dare to consider dousing Teddy Kennedy or Jesse Helms with a drink, despite the existence of more extreme provocation.

There were other incidents. One New Year's, about one-thirty in the morning as I remember, I called Bill Lynch of NBC to tell him what a lowlife degenerate he was, and how many years he would burn in hell because of a piece he had done for the network's year-end roundup. The show was still in progress when I made the call and was probably seen by at least three dozen people in the whole country, counting me.

I remember a similar conversation with Bob Pierpoint of CBS following an evening news piece. He had been out for the evening so I did not reach him until rather late. When I called him during the writing of this book for help in remembering what he had done to merit such a stern rebuke, he could not remember which of my profane phone calls I was talking about, much less the subject.

The point is that none of these incidents ever produced any repercussions, and I must say that I never felt that the way these reporters covered the next day's news was in the least affected by the events of the night before.

Which, come to think of it, is actually a little discouraging. Maybe I did not make my points clearly enough.

The final thing that appealed to me about journalists and journalism, then and now, was akin to what drew me to politics. At their best, both occupations are callings in the true sense of the word. Their ultimate end is public service. And the finest practitioners of journalism and politics are the sort of people who hold our battered, sometimes scruffy, democratic system together.

Many of the criticisms I have made and will make about journalists are equally applicable to public officials without changing a word. In the chapters that follow, as I rant and rave about unfair treatment of my former colleagues by the press, I hope the reader will not mistake my meaning. It is not that I object to politicians, particularly those at the national level, being held to a higher standard than other citizens. Much should be expected from those to whom much has been given.

But the fourth estate is also a privileged and elite institution. Journalists too have been given much by our society. There are those who argue that the First Amendment accords no more rights to reporters than to the average citizen, which sounds nice. But it isn't true. If you doubt that, try to get into a presidential press conference, or on the airplane that follows a President from Washington to Lagos and back, or even a transcript of a White House briefing, without a press pass.

I firmly believe that journalists also ought to be held to a higher standard, maybe not so high as Presidents and senators, but still higher than the rest of society. They ought to be, but they are not. The consequences of that laxity are what compose the balance of this book.

This brings me to one more thing I want to get on the record before we plunge into the trackless jungles of polemical denunciation and bitter recrimination.

I really liked my job. When you add it all up, I would not take anything in place of that opportunity. It always seemed at the time, and even more so now, to be a rare and wonderful privilege. It came my way not because I was the best-qualified person in the country to hold that particular position, but because I had the good fortune to be in the right place at the right time—and because of a President who was willing to give me a chance.

I cannot say the job was always pleasant, but it was certainly never, not even for a fleeting moment, boring.

To anyone who has ever dabbled in politics, the White House is Centre Court at Wimbledon, the World Cup, and the National Field Trials all rolled into one. It is where the stakes are the highest and the opportunities the greatest.

Like every other human that has ever lived, I look forward someday to being able to tell a grandchild about something I did that had a lasting and beneficial effect on somebody. Few places on earth provide as many chances to have the kind of effect on as many people as the White House.

Although it would be nice to take most, or even a good portion, of the credit for some momentous decision—on the Panama Canal treaties, or SALT, or Camp David accords, or energy legislation—I cannot do that.

About all I can say, come to think of it, is that there were occasions when good things were done that I could have screwed up, but did not. I am not sure exactly how one explains that sort of satisfaction to a grandchild; however, I am sure that a press secretary, even in his dotage, will retain some ability to put things in the best possible light.

Out of an abundance of caution, one further caveat should be included: this book is not intended to be an exhaustive compilation of every news story that I found distasteful. I do not want every story from those four years that is not mentioned in the pages that follow to be viewed as having cleared some sort of screening process. I have tried to touch upon the worst. It would take more than a single volume to set the record completely straight.

Some of those stories not included were unpleasant but accurate. Some were close enough calls to be not worth the trouble of explicating. Others were so technical and complex that getting at the "truth" of the matter in any reasonable number of pages is an impossibility. (Portions of the Bert Lance coverage that dealt with the nuances of the banking code fall into this category.) And there are a few that I still believe to be highly questionable, but I have been unable to prove, by any reasonable standard, to be as bad as I think they are.

It is possible that some, although I cannot imagine who, will be tempted to dismiss what follows as the rantings of an embittered press secretary. I plead guilty to having been a press secretary and to still being angry, if not embittered, about some of what I witnessed.

In the end, however, I hope the events and incidents I relate will be judged on their own merits. Was the journalism involved good or bad? To what extent were the mistakes excusable? And most important, do they add up to a situation that is serious enough to deserve careful scrutiny and our best efforts at improving?

You know already what my answer to all three of those questions would be. Being forewarned about my attitude should leave you armed with a sufficient degree of skepticism to proceed safely through the remainder of this book.

THE SCENE
OF THE CRIME_____

At 11:34 A.M. on January 20, 1981, I walked into the White House briefing room for my 1,245th and last briefing as White House press secretary. Unlike most of the others, this briefing was short, to the point, and there were no questions to be "taken" and dealt with later in the way. It was also an altogether fitting way for it all, or at least my part of it all, to end.

The press room was as packed for that final, less than earth-shaking announcement as it had been on numerous other occasions when a crisis somewhere in the world focused attention on the President of the United States and the aides, advisers, and support personnel who surrounded him. All of it has come to be referred to as the White House, a grammatically incorrect term for an institution that is both more and less than the President himself, or the government of the United States, or the executive branch.

I glanced briefly around the room, waiting the usual minute or two for conversation to cease and the inevitable few reporters caught on the phone in the back to hang up and race into the briefing room. I instinctively looked for familiar faces. There were a few. Those who would no longer be assigned to the White House, either by choice or because they had been replaced by a colleague who had covered the winning Reagan campaign, were there, along with a few who had been covering the Iran story so long from that briefing room that they just couldn't bear not to be there when it ended. The rest of the White House regulars were up on Capitol Hill, in effect already covering the President-elect, who would become the fortieth President of the United States in twenty-six minutes.

Within a few days after the election defeat in November, I had begun to think about appropriate parting comments for the White House regulars. I had even made a few notes and composed an outline of points I wanted to make, but this was neither the time nor the place. Time had run out on that idea, as it had on much else of much greater import that I and those who had come with me to the White House had planned or tried or dreamed of doing.

For those of us in the press office, it was, all things considered, a better way for it to end. We were busy up to the last moment. There was no time for recrimination or self-pity as the power and the spotlight shifted to the incoming administration. Psychologically, it helped to be working on little sleep and a lot of coffee as we had so many times before. Catching a short nap on the couch, slipping down to the basement of the West Wing for a quick shower, a shave, and a clean shirt, wives dropping in with a change of clothes. The familiar chaos, excitement, fatigue, and uncertainty were almost comforting.

I had not spent a night at home since Friday. Ruff Fant, my next-door neighbor, and Herky Harris, an old friend from Atlanta, had come down over the weekend to help haul away the boxes of memorabilia and personal papers. My wife and I had spent Saturday night in the Lincoln Bedroom. The invitation from President and Mrs. Carter had been primarily a thoughtful gesture, but also, I suspect, because the President knew this would be another long weekend and I would be sleeping somewhere in the White House anyway.

Most of the reporters and the press office staff had been on the job just as long or longer, without the benefit of even one comfortable and memorable night in Mr. Lincoln's bed. But they too would have had it no other way. The time had come to go, and this was the way to bid farewell.

And so in my last briefing, I simply told the press that there was no further word from Iran. Reports that the hostages were airborne, which had been flashing sporadically across the wire service machines since early that morning, were, unfortunately, false. I had to leave for Andrews Air Force Base to catch the plane back to Georgia with President Carter. Any further word on the impending release would have to come from the new administration.

Later, as we rode out to Andrews, listening halfheartedly to President Reagan's inaugural address, I reflected on how I had gotten into the press secretary business ten years before, almost by accident. Jimmy Carter had been in the process of winning an upset victory in the Democratic primary for governor of Georgia. His campaign press secretary was Bill Pope, a wise and irascible gentleman who loved and lived politics. But Pope cared less than nothing for the very different attractions of government office, and he had made it clear that his job ended on Election Day. I had no journalistic experience, but had gotten to know most of the political press in the state while traveling with the candidate, and I had become intrigued with them as individuals and as an institution. I had even begun to hope privately that if there was a place for me in the new administration it might be one that would allow me to continue to work with the press.

So I was surprised and delighted on election night when Governor-elect Carter offered not only a job in his administration, but the one job I most wanted but would never have requested: press secretary. I had neither the good judgment nor the good manners to demur even briefly.

Six years later, after an even more surprising election year, I had learned enough to talk seriously with the President-elect about whether he did not need someone a little older with Washington and journalism experience as his press secretary.

I had made the same argument at the beginning of that campaign in January of 1975. As he had then, the President-elect listened with a trace of a smile, undoubtedly knowing that I wanted the job despite my carefully constructed arguments to the contrary. At the end, he mentioned that he had thought about all my points, and he observed wryly that he was willing to take the risk if it would not be too great a sacrifice for me.

Once again, I accepted immediately.

So it came to pass, on the afternoon of inauguration day, I walked into the West Wing of the White House to go to work. Like almost every first-time visitor, I was impressed by how small it was. The halls are narrow, working areas cramped, meeting space limited, and the size of the entire West Wing staff less than one hundred. The press office is no exception, and it is impossible to begin to understand the relationship between the press and the White House without having some feel for the physical environment in which most of that interaction takes place.

When people speak of the White House Press Office, they usually mean the press office in the West Wing. That "office" is actually two offices, commonly referred to as the upper and lower press offices. The upper office, which occupies the northeast corner of the West Wing, contains the press secretary's office as well as offices for two deputies and cramped space for three secretaries.

The press secretary's office itself is the only spacious accommodation in either the upper or lower office. It is large enough for the press secretary to hold informal briefings for as many as twenty or twenty-five reporters. Once more than half again as large, it was reduced in size as part of extensive remodeling during the Johnson administration. Prior to that time, the daily briefings had been held in the press secretary's office because no briefing room existed and the White House press corps was small enough to be accommodated in a much smaller area.

A legacy of those years is the press secretary's desk. It is in the shape of half a horseshoe, effectively closing off one corner of the office and preventing inquisitive reporters from standing behind the press secretary and reading his notes or other confidential papers during briefings. It still serves this original purpose during informal sessions with reporters in the press secretary's office.

At the same time that the press secretary's office was reduced in size, it acquired heightened status by the addition of a fireplace, which sometimes provides the only cheery note, and always supplies ample quantities of smoke when the fire is not stoked to the conflagration level. Neglected fires in the press secretary's fireplace set off the White House smoke alarms so frequently that the sight of uniformed guards rushing into the upper press office became almost routine.

To get to the lower office, you walk east a few steps down a narrow corridor, turn left into a larger corridor, then turn right and go down a slight incline at a guard desk manned by a uniformed member of the Executive Protection Service. Then you make another left just before you reach a double set of glass doors that open onto the Rose Garden and the colonnade connecting the West Wing and the residence.

The lower office contains three small offices, one of which is a converted storage closet. Three desks and the press office Xerox machine are crowded together in a separate reception area, smaller than a modest hotel room.

That is it: a dozen staffers jammed into just over thirteen hundred square feet. There is additional office space for another two dozen or so people across West Executive Avenue in the Old Executive Office Building. But the principal burden of dealing with the White House press corps on a day-by-day, minute-by-minute basis falls on those twelve people.

If you walk east from the lower press office through a sliding wooden doorway, you leave the press office and enter the press room. Although technically a part of the West Wing, it is in fact the domain of the press corps. Both the press and the press office staff consider that door to be a line of demarcation. Both flow freely across it, in fact the press is allowed to roam over both the upper and the lower press offices, but both are aware of being on someone else's turf when they cross the line.

The White House press room is an unlikely-looking forum for great moments in history. It occupies the space above what was once the indoor swimming pool where some Presidents supposedly swam laps in the buff as they listened to briefings from aides. The pool is still there, but it was covered over by the Nixon administration to provide badly needed extra space for the White House press corps. It is the most informal and unkempt area of the White House, including the basement waiting room for White House drivers.

It is actually not one room, but three separate areas. The largest is the briefing room, 1,070 square feet, with a slightly raised platform and podium at the end adjacent to the lower press office, and a larger, partially screened platform for cameras at the other. It doubles as a lounge for waiting reporters and camera crews, and is thus usually littered with the remnants of snacks, cigar and cigarette butts, assorted papers of both an official and an unofficial nature, and miscellaneous pieces of camera and sound equipment. In my day, the furniture was a nondescript assortment of sofas and stuffed chairs, a television set, one table for eating and gambling, and a cluster of folding chairs grouped about the podium.

Soon after taking office, the Reagan administration decided to refurbish the press room. New pictures were hung, new carpet installed, and eight rows of six chairs each implanted in front of the podium. The primary purpose was to encourage greater decorum during the press secretary's briefings. It was hoped that a more orderly and less informal physical arrangement would promote a similar change in the behavior of the reporters in attendance.

The original redesign by the Nixon administration, which included the construction of the raised stage and podium, was also intended to promote a more respectful audience. Neither effort had, nor could have had, more than a transient and limited impact.

Behind the briefing room is the press working area. On your right as you enter from the briefing room are two enclosed booths of precisely equal dimensions for the Associated Press and United Press International. Next are three rows of carrels, about the size of those provided to graduate students at a medium-size university whose new library has not yet been completed. These are assigned to print reporters who cover the White House on a regular basis by the White House Press Office.

On rare occasions when one of these carrels becomes vacant, the decision on which of the waiting news organizations will receive it is always traumatic. Angry letters, appeals, and protests flood the press office. Occasionally legal action is threatened. Finally, a decision is made and the whole thing is forgotten in about two days.

Just off to the left of the working area is another smaller area containing vending machines, indifferently stocked and serviced, a refrigerator donated *in memoriam* by the widow of a White House correspondent, restrooms, and another combination snack and gin table.

Across the back of the working area are arrayed the networks in semisoundproof picture-window booths, only slightly larger than those occupied by the wire services at the other end.

Beneath the working area is a room with small booths for radio correspondents, even smaller carrels for writers, and a water cooler. Reporters assigned to this area, which they refer to as the dungeon, live in constant terror that a White House staffer or distinguished visitor will wander into the briefing room to conduct an impromptu press conference. There is a public address system for announcing briefings and the posting of printed material, but it is seldom used for these casual sessions. Visitors will often break off a session if it is announced, and White House staff members who drop by to peddle some tidbit of information do not want the informality of their pitch jeopardized by an announcement. As a result, press office staffers in the lower office are beseeched by reporters in the basement to slip down with a word of warning whenever news is being made quietly in the briefing room.

The physical proximity of press room and press office combines with the cramped space in the press office to produce a physical intimacy that parallels the psychological closeness of the relationship.

The lower press office is almost always awash with reporters checking on when a transcript will be ready, what time the President will be leaving for Camp David that weekend, what time the press secretary will brief, or just gossiping with the staff. When big news is breaking, the upper office also becomes packed with waiting and sometimes impatient reporters. At times the crowd becomes so large that it is almost impossible for the secretaries to function and reporters are asked to clear the upper press office area.

More often, they are allowed to stay. The turmoil and distractions become a familiar part of the environment. Those who leave the press office for jobs in private enterprise, or even other areas of government, sometimes find they have a hard time working in the quieter, more decorous surroundings.

More to the point, reporters are allowed to stay because of a shared sense of participation in what is happening. In many cases, the press office, indeed the whole White House, is awaiting the next development with the same anticipation as the press. At those times of crisis and pivotal decision the press gravitates emotionally and physically toward the President and the Oval Office. The upper press office is as close as they can get, and the press office staff is as reluctant to banish them to the briefing room as they would be to go there themselves.

Times of crisis are also the occasions when the work environment for press staff and press is most similar. Normally, the pace of work is quite different.

The White House beat can be extremely frustrating for a reporter. It is confining. It tends not to reward hard work or initiative nearly as much as other assignments. On most days the difference between a smart, experienced, hard-driving reporter and one who is just the opposite will not be reflected in their work. A typical reporter's day is characterized by long stretches of boredom interrupted by intense activity and pressure.

For the press staff, boredom is never a problem. If the importance of events is not adequate, the very multitude of them will keep the pressure on, without respite. The press staff spends a great portion of its time collecting, checking, and preparing information for presentation to the press. The longer this process of preparation takes, the later the press will receive the information, the closer will be their deadlines, and the more intense will be the pressure on them.

This juxtaposition of reporters looking for something to do and staffers desperately searching for the time to catch up with work they should have done yesterday is one cause of tension between the two groups. It is usually handled with reasonably good nature, except when reporters believe, usually but not always incorrectly, that they are being intentionally "jammed" by the press office. That expression refers to the gambit of delaying a controversial or unpleasant statement in an attempt to reduce both the attention it receives and the time the press has to follow up and to punch holes in the administration's arguments.

This combination of proximity, tension, personalities, varying levels of mutual understanding and suspicion, and the constant knowledge that both institutions need one another produces a unique environment. It is unlike any other in government or anywhere else, to my knowledge.

I came to the White House with so little in the way of expectations that it was hard to be surprised. I had taken time during the transition period between election and inauguration to talk at length with almost all former White House press secretaries. Democrats and Republicans alike, they were unfailingly generous with their time and candid with their advice, and they warned to a man that there was no such thing as being well prepared for the job.

As it turned out, their advice, which I continued to seek throughout the four years, was always more valuable than they thought. Almost as helpful was the chance to talk to someone who understood the problems I was facing as only one who has been there can. (Having brought them into this book early, I suppose I ought to say that it goes without saying that they and their counsel can in no way be held responsible for my sins of omission and commission.)

As I talked with them and with others, including some in the press, and as I lived through my four years in the White House, I came to the conclusion that this relationship between Presidents and press was both more important than was generally understood, and less well understood than it generally should be.

For almost a decade, the impression of the presidency as a troubled institution has been growing. Attention has focused on and much has been written about the relationship of the presidency to the Congress, the courts, the bureaucracy, political parties, and the changes in our society as a whole. Much less has been said about the relationship of the presidency to one of the most powerful institutions in our society, the press.

I have always believed that the primary responsibility of a President is leadership—to move, shape, and direct the expression of popular will through our system of government. That is, to take the long view and to take the country a little further than or not quite so fast as it is naturally inclined to go. That, to me, is the guts of it all.

There are other important roles: personification of the nation and the national will, leadership of a political party, even satisfaction of that supposed craving of the American people for some sort of quasi-monarch. However, I suspect this particular job description was primarily the invention of politicians who wanted to live like kings, in cahoots with the academicians, who fancied themselves as advisers to princes rather than democrats.

That ability to make us lift our eyes above both the passions and indifference of the moment, to some common vision of our future welfare as individuals and as a nation, is almost totally dependent upon the workings of the relationship between press and President.

To paraphrase one who knew a great deal about changing and lifting the vision of people: How shall they believe in what they have not heard? How shall they hear without a preacher?

And if Saint Paul had worked in the White House, he surely would have added, "How shall the preacher be heard, except through the press?"

Forget about the vaunted ability of a modern President to speak directly to the nation on prime-time television, or at least put it into perspective. It is a powerful tool, but extremely limited. President Carter made public comments about matters of concern to the nation on more than 1,451 different occasions for a cumulative total of 437 hours and 38 minutes. But only 35 of those occasions and 17 hours and 51 minutes were broadcast live during prime time. All the rest was heard through the press. That, in itself, is neither good nor bad; it is just the way things work.

For the most part, what we know about, or think we know about, our accumulated total of facts and impressions about the most important questions of government action and policy, depends neither on "what the press tells us" nor on what the President says. The theory of a monolithic, conspiring, biased press and the myth of an all-powerful, manipulative, unchecked President are inaccurate, not even serviceable heuristic devices. Neither institution has anything that approaches total control over what we see, hear, and read. What we get, what we depend upon, is the product of a dynamic, confusing, unceasing interaction— the relationship between President and press.

By the end of four years in the White House, I had reached the conclusion that this relationship between the press and the presidency is seriously flawed. It fails to provide the President with an adequate channel for communicating with, for moving, shaping, and directing the popular will. Perhaps more important, it also fails to provide the nation with the quantity and quality of reasonably accurate information its citizens need to make the decisions necessary for self-government.

That opinion has been modified somewhat during the researching and writing of this book, but it has not been basically changed.

The reasons the relationship does not work very well relate to both institutions, the White House and the press. And the problems go much more to the impersonal, institutional pressures that constrain those who work in the White House and those who cover the White House. There is also a striking similarity between the pressures faced by both groups.

Both a President and his aides and the White House reporters operate against artificially imposed deadlines that may or may not have anything to do with the pace of events in the real world. And both are forced to deal not only with their own deadlines but with those of the other institution as well.

Both institutions routinely make decisions based upon inadequate, sometimes woefully inadequate, information. This is true not only because of deadline pressures and the problems of collecting and processing the available information. It is most often true because both institutions deal frequently with questions for which the answers are essentially unknowable, at least in any empirical sense. (I mean to say here not only that the answers are not knowable "immediately" but that they are not determinable in any empirical sense ever. A good part of history is the continuing argument over whether governmental decisions over past years were correct. The reason the argument continues is that there is no answer that can be proven to be the right one. We still do not know with certainty and never will.) These questions are, in the term of the trade, judgment calls. In such situations even if all the hard information could be collected, which it never can, and even if there were all the time in the world to analyze it, which there never is, reasonable and intelligent individuals would differ.

The above happens also to be a good description of the so-called presidential decision—that question which will have to be answered by the President because of its importance and because the call is so close that presidential authority must be invoked. That is the realm in which the White House lives. Those who cover it must operate within those boundaries.

Both elements react to and make decisions based upon rather dimly perceived ideas of what the other is doing or about to do. It was not uncommon to find myself at midmorning trying to determine where the press was heading on a particularly important story. If they appeared to be off by 15 degrees to the right of what we thought was accurate, we would craft a statement that would administer a 15-degree course correction back to the left. By the time the statement was issued in the early afternoon briefing, we sometimes found them heading off by 15 degrees in the opposite direction. Our carefully honed statement served not to correct but to exacerbate.

For its part, the press sometimes becomes so fascinated with interpretations of what the President *did not* say, or how he did or did not say it, or what he really meant, that they miss the point of what he actually did say and what that clearly meant.

Both institutions face an increasingly skeptical, even hostile public. Neither is held in particularly high regard by those it is supposed to serve, and the problem for both threatens to get worse over the long haul rather than better.

Both institutions also have a tendency to become overly defensive when under attack. The "circle the wagons; everyone is out to get us" syndrome in the White House is a generally familiar problem. The "circle the typewriters; the First Amendment is at stake" phenomenon in the press is at least as common, almost as serious in its consequences, and much less well recognized or understood.

Finally, both institutions, partially as a result of the tendency toward paranoia, fail to punish adequately mistakes and incompetence. The consequences of this shortcoming are perhaps more serious in the press than in the White House, not because reporters are necessarily more prone to error, but because the political process, of which the press is an important part, works to expose and punish mistakes in government. There is for the press no system of external discipline that is even remotely comparable.

Having listed some of the problems, which will be expanded on and illustrated in the remainder of this book, a writer has at least some obligation to suggest what should be done. There is a temptation to adopt the approach of Will Rogers, who once advised President Wilson on how to deal with the problem of German U-boats:

"Just bring the Atlantic Ocean to a boil," Rogers said; "I'll leave the details to the technicians."

But one could argue that the Republic has more to fear from the press–White House relationship than it ever has had from submarines. So, I shall provide some ideas on what must be done in the concluding chapters.

POLITICAL BIAS:
THE SCREWBALL SPIN__

The research shows that most reporters are Democrats, and liberal Democrats at that. But what does that mean for a Democratic President? The answer is not necessarily what one might expect. To the extent that left-of-center political or ideological preferences are a factor in what reporters (as opposed to columnists or commentators) say and write, it cuts two ways.

Part of the problem is the somewhat incestuous relationship between journalism and government that still exists in Washington. It occurs elsewhere too. The relationships of local papers and TV stations with the political and economic establishment are certainly not unknown in towns small and large around the country. But it is different in Washington. For one thing, most news organizations that indulge in this sort of thing elsewhere are more up-front about it. They will even defend it as being good for the state or the city.

In Washington, though, nobody ever admits to anything, particularly not the press. As a result, the problem is a lot more complicated and harder to get a grip on.

The way this relates to Democratic reporters and Democratic Presidents has to do both with expectations—the standards reporters apply to Presidents—and with access to information—what is available to them to use in enforcing those standards.

First, let us deal with the expectations. Those journalists who really care about certain policy positions tend to hold Democratic Presidents to a higher standard. They don't expect Republicans to do much for women or minorities or poor people, and they don't raise much hell when they don't. They expect Republicans to be a good bit laxer about conflicts of interest and other improprieties and don't pursue such stories, at least since Watergate, with as much zeal in a GOP administration.

Thus, you have the strange situation of Mr. Reagan catching less hell from this quarter for chopping away at social programs than did Mr. Carter for cutting the rate of increase in payments. And you see the same journalists who scorched Bert Lance for bank overdrafts that took place years before he came into government grinning and shuffling while William Casey, with access to the most highly classified economic information in the world, traded massively in the stock market.

This double standard on the part of the more liberal thinkers in the press is reinforced by the same sort of psychology among interest groups. They know very well that most Republican Presidents, particularly Mr. Reagan, don't give a damn what they think, say, or do. So they are inclined to clam up and be less active, thus giving the press less critical material to work with.

President Carter used to meet every couple of months with the Congressional Black Caucus, for example. As a result, he was subjected to public excoriation by the caucus leadership following every meeting, usually from the front steps of the White House, because he would not agree to everything they wanted.

President Reagan, who wouldn't touch the black caucus with his riding quirt, much less see them out through the front door, has been the object of much less abuse.

The behavior of some of the national women's groups was, if anything, worse. Their reaction to Carter, who agreed with them on most things except federal funding of abortion, was to chain themselves to the White House fence. Logic would dictate that their reaction to Mr. Reagan would be something close to self-immolation in Lafayette Park, an event that, fortunately or unfortunately, depending on your point of view, has yet to take place.

At no time was this screwball attitude better demonstrated than during and after the 1980 Democratic convention. Prominent leaders of the women's movement, including Gloria Steinem and Eleanor Smeal, then president of the National Organization for Women, professed to be quite unable to determine whether Ronald Reagan or Jimmy Carter would be a better President for women. They seemed to think that independent candidate John Anderson, whose only possible impact was to aid in the election of Mr. Reagan, might be the source of salvation.

I observed at the time that if they ended up with Ronald Reagan they would soon find out and would richly deserve what they got. They now have him, have presumably learned the answer to their quandary of 1980, and there is a large element of justice in it all—for them, if not for the women of this country who suffer from discrimination and who depended on them for leadership. (To be fair, it should be said that not all the leaders of all women's organizations were so shortsighted.)

But it also should be noted that Ronald Reagan has proven to be a financial blessing for NOW. Their contribution to his election has been repaid by policies that have resulted in an increased flow of contributions to their coffers amounting to millions of dollars over the past three years. In that sense, life is truly unfair.

Now we come to the information part of the problem—what the press has to work with—which also has two pieces. In the first place, the reporters know more about the intricacies of liberal proposals: they have followed them more closely because of personal as well as professional interests. Those who draft and advocate various items of the liberal agenda are more likely to be the friends and associates of these journalists. As a result, the journalists understand and have great access to the nuances and legislative histories of various sections, subsections, and alternatives. And so, like novelists who are happiest writing about the things they know most about, they will quibble with and niggle to death a Democratic President who supports the principles of something like national health insurance or arms control or nuclear nonproliferation, but differs on tactics and timing—while being less nasty to a Republican, who is totally opposed to the whole idea.

The other part of the information problem—which you will remember was a part of the bias problem—has to do with the behavior of people in government. Those who support particular policies are much more inclined to take their gripes, complaints, and tips to a sympathetic reporter. As a result, Democratic Presidents are more bedeviled by leaks than Republicans.

If you are a staffer on the Hill, or in some agency of the

executive branch, and you have a career invested in a particular approach to arms control or national health insurance—an approach not endorsed in every detail by the President—there will be no difficulty in finding a number of reporters who understand and sympathize with your pet project. They will be eager to construct a story based on your gripes about the ineptitude and/or lack of sincere commitment on the part of the crypto-Republican crackers in the White House.

Meanwhile, columnists and commentators are subject to the same sort of expectations and information pressures. But the consequences are even more unfortunate.

In the first place, columnists and commentators have greater latitude because they are dealing in opinion, unconstrained by rules of objective news reporting that tend to take the edge off the worst biases among reporters.

In addition, the information differential has greater impact on columnists because they normally do not work as hard as reporters and thus have to make what little information they have go further. (I can personally attest to the above, having been in the column-writing business for the past two years.)

The nature of the business also tends to push column writers toward political extremes to an even greater extent than it does reporters. The pressure is to be provocative, to have a point of view, even to be outrageous.

Most presidential decisions are close calls, very much of this-on-the-one-hand-and-that-on-the-other type. Most columns and commentaries are not. The result is unfortunate for any President of the moderate center, be he Democrat or Republican. It is easy to list columnists who write from the point of view of the Democratic left: Tom Wicker, Mary McGrory, Tony Lewis, and the like. The list on the right includes Evans and Novak, George Will, and James Kilpatrick. Compiling a list of those consistently in the center is extremely difficult.

Jack Anderson may be considered nonideological, but hardly moderate or centrist. In the great tradition of divinely inspired writers, he is certainly beyond partisanship. His *modus operandi* is to take care of those who will feed him dirt on others, and flail away at everyone else without regard to ideology or accuracy.

In the 1980 presidential campaign, we ran into a peculiar and painful example of how the political preferences of journalists can have an impact that is exactly the reverse of what one might expect.

What happened, if the statements of the reporters themselves can be credited, was the result of three factors:

First, they overcompensated for their ideological preferences. Knowing that they disagreed with Reagan's positions, they went out of their way not to be overly critical of them in their reporting, and to be particularly skeptical of what Carter had to say.

Second, they were worried about the allegations that the "eastern liberal press" was always unfair to candidates from the right. Their concerns dated back to the Goldwater campaign of 1964, when any objective observer would have had to conclude that Goldwater did receive rougher treatment than Johnson. This time they were going to prove that they could be "fair" to a right-winger, no matter what. In consequence, as many would admit later, they were more than fair. Candidate Reagan was often allowed to slip off the hook when he made statements and proposals that would have produced a firestorm had they issued from any other presidential candidate.

More to the point, his statements were not mere slips of the tongue, or unfortunate choices of words that unintentionally distorted his true meaning. They were just the opposite: clear indications of his true intentions, of what he planned to do if elected, and has done for the past three years.

Finally, many of the reporters who covered the White House had decided by the time the 1980 campaign rolled around that they personally did not like Carter. Some now argue that this opinion was fully justified, but few maintain that it did not exist. The result of this personal antipathy was to make their overcompensation in favor of Mr. Reagan easier for them to live with.

Three examples of the way this set of attitudes operated to the President's detriment come to mind.

On October 6, 1980, the President was in West Allis, Wisconsin. His major speech of the day was an attack on Reaganomics. The theme was that Reagan's proposals to slash taxes, to cut or eliminate domestic programs while "shifting responsibilities to the states," and to greatly increase defense expenditures would place great pressure on state and local budgets, and thus increase the more regressive sales and property taxes that financed them.

A copy of the President's speech was distributed on the press plane before landing in Milwaukee. No sooner had I arrived at the first event than I was informed by an aide that Lou Cannon of the *Washington Post* had spent most of the flight out trying to convince other reporters on the plane that Carter's attack on Reagan was inaccurate and unfair. It was, according to Cannon, certainly a misinterpretation of Reagan's proposals and possibly an international exercise in demagogy.

I lost no time in accosting Cannon, who had covered Reagan for years from the *Post*'s West Coast bureau and was known to be close to him and his people. Was he, I inquired heatedly, a reporter or a Reagan campaign aide? We had carefully researched the figures that supported our charges. If he had specific questions about them, I wanted to hear them now.

As the rest of the traveling press corps looked on, Cannon reiterated his defense of the Reagan proposals. He did not raise questions about the numbers; he just felt that, based on his years of experience covering Mr. Reagan, it would be a mistake to assume that his statements on such matters should be taken literally. We were, he said again, being unfair, interpreting the campaign proposals to suit our own purposes.

It quickly became obvious to me that I was losing the argument. My numbers and the facts carried little weight in the face of Cannon's determined charges of distortion and in the context of a White House press corps that had already decided Carter was being "mean" and "unfair." (More on that later.)

Fearing another round of stories that accused the President of mean-spirited and demogogic attacks on his opponent, I suggested to the President that he change his speech, which was not to be delivered until several hours later. He did so, softening his attacks on the Reagan policies. The result was that they received little attention from print or broadcast media. We were, indeed, never able to focus the campaign discourse on the consequences of Reaganomics.

In retrospect, I should have disregarded Cannon's arguments and the quick acceptance of them by his colleagues. They would at least have been forced to report what the President had said, even if they had attempted to denigrate them while doing so. The consequences for the Carter campaign could hardly have been worse in the long run.

There would also have been at least some historical satisfaction. The effects of Reaganomics on local governments and taxpayers have been very close to what was predicted in the text that Mr. Cannon found so unfair. Those results would have been even more painful had the Congress not rejected his proposals for a "New Federalism" for many of the reasons presented in that text.

The other incidents occurred when the press allowed Mr. Reagan to escape the normal consequences of his own actions involving what we had come to refer to as the war and peace issue. It was his greatest liability throughout the campaign. Many Americans thought Carter was not tough enough in dealing with our potential adversaries. But at least an equal number were worried that Mr. Reagan's belligerent and occasionally cavalier attitude about the use of military force might be an even more immediate and serious danger. These concerns focused primarily, although not exclusively, on nuclear weapons and the threat of nuclear war.

On January 31, 1980, in Jacksonville, Florida, Mr. Reagan delivered himself of the startling observation that he did not think the proliferation of nuclear weapons was "any of our business." He then criticized the efforts of the Carter administration to halt the spread of such devices and technology, implying that such foolishness would have no place in a Reagan administration (as indeed it has not).

When we saw the reports of this startling observation moving across the wires, we were delighted. The Gipper had really stepped in it now. The idea of nuclear weapons in the hands of a madman like Muammar Qaddafi or Idi Amin, or any number of other unbalanced leaders around the world, was a danger that most Americans could easily understand. Nor were such fears groundless. Most experts in the area are convinced that a nuclear exchange is more likely to come as the result of the actions of some smaller country than through intentional acts or miscalculation on the part of the superpowers.

Our jubilation was short-lived. The Reagan staff recognized that danger immediately and set about trying to limit the damage.

Without much hope of success by their own admission, they trotted the candidate out an hour later to try to explain away his comments.

What he meant, the governor said, was that the nonproliferation efforts of the Carter administration had been ineffective. They had been pursued so ineptly that the results had been more harm than good in our relations with our allies and with emerging third-world countries.

Now that was a decent political argument, incorrect in our view, but up to us to ignore or disprove. However, it was not in any way similar to what Reagan had first said. He had not questioned the implementation of the policy, but the policy itself. Even in his clarification session, he repeated the earlier none-of-our-business remark. And as the actions of his administration would later show, he meant exactly what he said.

The press, for the most part, swallowed the "explanation" and shrugged off what the candidate had actually said. None of the three networks mentioned the "I don't think nuclear proliferation is any of our business" comment. Nor did the print media evidence any great excitement over the fact that the frontrunner for the GOP nomination wanted to get the U.S. government out of the nonproliferation business. The *Washington Post* led with Reagan's charge that Carter's policies were "increasing the risk of nuclear war," brushing by the nonproliferation statement in two lines in the bottom third of the story.

Our attempts to revive the issue during the fall campaign were met by sublime indifference on the part of the press. We were just looking for something to dredge up in the hope that it would distract attention from our own problems. Hadn't the whole thing been satisfactorily explained right away? Wasn't this just another example of Carter and his people trying to portray that nice Mr. Reagan as some sort of crazy?

The net result was that a statement that would have bedeviled any other candidate for days—try to imagine the reaction if Humphrey, Nixon, McGovern, or Ford, not to mention Carter, had spouted such idiocy—disappeared from sight. When we referred to it after Mr. Reagan became the nominee, most voters and a large number of reporters did not even know what we were talking about.

An equally startling comment from Mr. Reagan and reaction from the press occurred a few months later, right in the middle of the fall campaign. In a lengthy interview with the Associated Press, candidate Reagan described in some detail how he would handle arms control negotiations with the Soviet Union. The one card that had not been played, he said, was the threat of an "all-out nuclear arms race." And if he was elected President, he suggested, that option would be a real one.

Once again we were ecstatic. That was just the sort of thing that worried voters about Reagan. The cost and the dangers associated with such a policy were easy to document and easy for voters to understand. Although our enthusiasm was tempered somewhat by our bitter experience with the proliferation episode, we were sure that no candidate for the presidency would ever be allowed to get away with two such inanities on such an important issue in the same campaign.

Though the quote was buried in the story on the interview, so had been Carter's famous comment about ethnic purity four years earlier. I was sure that it would not remain buried for long. We jumped on it immediately, calling it to the attention of reporters and arranging public statements condemning such dangerous talk from a host of prominent Democrats.

The entire effort was wasted. The arms race quote was given even less attention by the press than the nonproliferation quote. The networks ignored it totally, although they found eight minutes for generally positive coverage of the Anderson campaign; and the print media did not do much better. This time the Reagan people, who had winced when they read the quote, did not even have to bother with trying to explain it away.

Once again the actions of the Reagan administration have conformed precisely to the comments he made on the campaign trail, comments that we could not persuade anyone in the press to see as being significant.

All of this was both cause and part of what came to be known as the meanness issue in the campaign. It was one of the classic cases in which the press becomes not a medium of information, but a powerful actor—deciding for itself what the public ought to think about what is going on and then acting to turn that "ought to" into reality.

The meanness issue was the belief on the part of a number of influential journalists that Jimmy Carter was being mean and unfair and ugly to Ronald Reagan, just as he had been mean and unfair to Teddy Kennedy earlier in the year. Not only did these journalists decide that Carter was being mean, which was their perfect right as citizens, they also decided that this was a significant political issue, meaning that the electorate was or should have been interpreting the President's behavior in the same way as the journalists.

It was, from start to finish, all in their heads. Although there were certainly cases of rhetorical excess from the President and the rest of us in the Carter camp, they were hardly more extravagant than what was emerging from the Reagan campaign. The press, presumably for the reasons mentioned earlier in this chapter, chose to focus its attention and criticism solely on the Carter statements.

Despite the extra coverage that the Carter comments received, the available polling data showed that if meanness was a political issue, its impact on the public was exactly the opposite of what the press was preaching. Less than 40 percent of the voters thought either candidate was being "mean," and by a margin of four to one *they* thought the mean candidate was Mr. Reagan.

Eventually it got so bad that the President could hardly say anything that was critical of his opponent without his rhetoric becoming more of an issue than the substance of his remarks. We decided that we had to find some way to get this thing behind us—not because the voters were exercised about it (the polls still showed that of those who thought anybody was running a mean campaign, most thought it was Reagan), but because we had to be able to make an issue of the positions and proposals coming from our opponent. We clearly could not survive a campaign in which we were constantly on the defensive.

It was a frustrating business. The President was not particularly eager to apologize for something that no one except a few journalists thought he was any more guilty of than his opponent. And I did not blame him for his reluctance. Nevertheless, something had to be done.

We finally settled on an interview with Barbara Walters, who had been requesting one for several weeks. With the request came a promise that it would be shown on the evening news, which guaranteed wide distribution, and that we would get three to four minutes, thus helping to ensure that the President would have time to say what he wanted to say in his own words.

The President did an admirable job, not quite apologizing, but admitting that he had been excessively harsh on occasions while maintaining that the other side had been at least as guilty. He expressed the hope that we could get beyond this issue and promised to do his part.

As grating as it was to have to do, the interview worked—for about two days. Then in Florida he made so bold as to suggest that the election of Mr. Reagan would be a "bad thing" for the country and that he didn't think he would be a "good President" or a "good man to trust with the affairs of the nation." That was hardly a brutal or even a surprising assessment of a political opponent, but the press was quickly back into its "meanness" frenzy.

At the time I thought the President was indeed guilty of occasional hyperbole; looking back on it now I am less critical of some of his comments. The remark that most reporters say kicked the whole issue off was a warning that the election of Ronald Reagan would divide the nation "rich from poor, black from white, Jew from Christian, North from South, rural from urban." Certainly with regard to the first two categories, the President's prediction was right on the mark. The other basis for the "meanness" charge was Carter's warning that Mr. Reagan was so inclined to rely upon military force that he might "lead us into war." That, of course, is a ridiculous idea, and no one these days thinks that anything like that could ever happen. At worst, Carter's rhetoric was no worse than campaign commercials being run by Reagan supporters charging the President with being in favor of putting homosexuals in the classrooms of elementary schools across the land, and of being a declared enemy of the American family.

Although President Carter readily admits to a weakness for hyperbole and the superlative, I have always believed that at least a part of his tendency in that direction during the '80 campaign was a result of massive frustration. We had been unable to get the press to pay any attention whatsoever to Reagan's nonsensical statements or even to the consequences of what his major policy positions might be. When Vice-President Walter Mondale tried to draw attention to such things, as he did with regard to the nuclear nonproliferation and the "all-out arms race" episodes, he was ignored. Attempts by the press office or others associated with the campaign to draw attention to them were like spitting into a hurricane.

Still it would have been better had the President been a bit more subtle in his efforts—a rapier rather than a machete might have been more effective. I say might have because I have some doubt whether there was in fact a workable approach for us with the press by that time. It is very likely, I think, that anything subtle enough not to be called mean or demagogic would have been too subtle for the press to cover, as per the toned-down attack on Reaganomics mentioned earlier.

Whatever the causes, we never quite got out from under the issue again. It was the context in which Reagan's "There you go again" rejoinder in the debate was so effective. The press, with some help from us, had managed to open a nice hole for the Gipper, and he waltzed right through it for a touchdown!

THE MISSING
PLANE

I believe that our relations with the press began to fray in the late summer of 1977, when the prolonged and painful dispute over allegations against Bert Lance, the President's budget director, led to hard feelings on both sides. I became emotionally involved in Bert's defense. My frustration and bitterness grew as it became increasingly clear to me that he could not survive the controversy.

On the morning of September 13, 1977, the papers were filled with negative stories about Lance. The morning shows featured clips of senators, including Charles Percy of Illinois, proclaiming their outrage at the recent revelation that Lance had used a plane owned by his bank to fly to University of Georgia football games.

A few days earlier, a Chicago businessman had mentioned to a White House staffer that Percy was in no position to be talking, because he had regularly used a corporation plane, owned by Bell and Howell, which he formerly headed, to fly back and forth to Washington. The staffer had passed the information on to me. I was tempted at the time to give the tip to a reporter or two, but decided against it.

On the morning of the thirteenth, however, I changed my mind. The consequences were disastrous.

I called several reporters and told them what I had heard. One of them was Loye Miller, then Washington bureau chief for the *Chicago Sun-Times*. The next morning, on the front page of the *Sun-Times* there was a story describing how I had launched an "offensive aimed at discrediting" a United States senator—including a reference to my description of Senator Percy as a "sanctimonious SOB." The *Sun-Times* reported that it had checked into my "allegations" about corporate plane trips and found them to be false.

I was sick and outraged. In my view, I had been passing on an off-the-record tip—a common practice in Washington—never claiming that I could verify its accuracy. That was up to the reporters. (Loye claims that I never explicitly said that my tip was off the record, so he felt justified in revealing his source and writing about the incident.)

But my embarrassment was the least important consideration. I had damaged Bert's case by a thoughtless action. The first task was to limit the damage.

I went immediately to explain the situation to the President. On my way to the Oval Office, Frank Moore told me he had heard that Percy was planning to take the floor of the Senate to denounce my actions.

To say that the President was unhappy is an understatement. I told him that the only thing I could think of to do was to call Percy and apologize and then take my lumps from the press. He agreed.

Within five minutes, I had Percy on the phone. He was most gracious in accepting my apology, and said that as far as he was concerned, that was the end of it.

I then called Bert to apologize for what I had done to him and to let him know what Percy had said. Bert did his best to make me feel better, but he and I both knew that the incident had hurt him badly.

Shortly thereafter, I told a packed briefing room that I considered my behavior to have been "irresponsible, stupid, and wrong" and that the President agreed with that characterization.

That night the evening news broadcasts presented the whole sorry mess to the country, complete with commentary from Loye Miller. Two networks made it their lead story with references to Watergate-style "dirty tricks." The next day, the *Sun-Times* bannered my apology across the top of page 1.

I had made two mistakes. It was indeed stupid of me to have involved myself in such an enterprise. If the tip was worth some reporter's time to check out—and considering what I knew about the source, it seemed to be—it should have been passed on by someone other than the President's press secretary.

To make matters worse, I had called in Loye Miller, a reporter who was known by many—but not by me—to be as close to Percy as any journalist in Washington. As a new boy in town, I had tripped over my unfamiliarity with the Washington terrain— and tripped badly. You just do not give potentially damaging information about a politician to a reporter who is known to be close to him. The reporter may not use it, out of fear of destroying a productive relationship; if he does use it, the story is likely to read somewhat differently from what you had in mind, although seldom as differently as this one.

However, as it turns out, mine was not the only mistake. Years later while researching this book, I happened to be talking to Andrew Glass, Washington bureau chief for Cox Newspapers, who was one of the other reporters I had called on that unfortunate morning. (Unbeknownst to me at the time of that first call, and as further evidence of my pitiful lack of information about Washington, Andy had once worked for several years as Senator Percy's administrative assistant.) Toward the close of our conversation, Andy said there was something I should know.

There had been a plane, and Senator Percy had frequently used it to travel between Illinois and Washington. The plane was owned not by Bell and Howell but by Motorola. Although there was nothing illegal about the practice, and this was well before such behavior by public officials began to be questioned, Andy and some other members of the senator's staff became concerned about the propriety of the trips. After much discussion, Glass said, the senator reluctantly agreed to pay the price of a commercial airline ticket for each trip.

Later, Glass said, he discovered that the senator's checks were not being cashed. He was bothered by this and raised the point, but, as he was about to leave the staff, did not follow up on it. He does not know how it was finally resolved.

Andy had neither said nor written anything about what he knew at the time of the flap, because he considered it improper to use something he had heard as a senator's staffer against him. An understandable position. I assumed he was telling me now, knowing that I was writing a book, to set the record straight.

When all is said and done, none of this alters the fact that I made a serious mistake in the way I handled the matter. If questions remain, they relate to the possibility that reporters can get too close to politicians for their own good. Loye Miller was apparently misled, if not deceived, by Senator Percy's office. But in one sense he asked for it. Whether he would have accepted their denial so readily had he maintained more of an arm's length relationship only he can judge.

CAMPAIGNING FOR PEACE___

The search for peace and stability in the Middle East was a priority for the Carter administration from beginning to end. There were stops and starts, ups and downs—some missed opportunities, and great progress that came from seizing or creating opportunities where none seemed to exist. The amount of press coverage generated by this campaign with its numerous meetings between heads of state and governments was commensurate with the emphasis placed on it by the President.

For the purposes of a book about White House–press relationships, there are two focal points that offer several lessons about the interaction between the two institutions: the Camp David summit, which took place from September 5 through September 17 of 1978, and President Carter's trip to Cairo and Jerusalem, which lasted from March 7 to March 15 of the following year.

The result of those two efforts, and of the months of meetings, negotiations, plans, and schemes before, after, and in between, was a peace treaty between Israel and Egypt and a plan for the creation of an autonomous Palestinian entity composed of the West Bank of the Jordan and the Gaza Strip.

At this writing, the peace treaty, although strained and battered, still prevents the outbreak of another major war in that region. The plan for Palestinian autonomy has gone nowhere. It has been the victim of not so benign neglect during the first eighteen months of the Reagan administration, Israeli intransigence, and criminally shortsighted leadership in the Arab world, particularly among the Palestinians.

When the treaty was signed, in March of 1979, the President received little credit for his accomplishments. Indeed, the entire Middle East peace effort, taken as a whole, was decidedly a net minus for Jimmy Carter politically. Part of that was the result of the interconnection between the problems of the region and the American political process. But part of it was also due to the way the President's efforts were covered in the press, particularly in their final stages.

Unfortunately for the President I served, the culmination of what was perhaps his greatest diplomatic accomplishment came at a time when the press corps was largely unwilling to give him credit for much of anything. It was a time when I used to say that if the First Lady had conceived, the White House press corps would have declared that it had happened despite the President's best efforts.

My attitude about those who displayed the greatest animus has not changed. Nor, apparently, has theirs. As this book was being completed, syndicated columnist Joseph Kraft, one of the strangest sorts of a peculiar breed, was moved to observe in relation to the most recent difficulties in the region that Carter's diplomatic triumph had been "almost mindlessly reached."

The press and communications setting for these two events could not have been more dissimilar. The Camp David summit took place in relative isolation, on American soil, after ample opportunity for planning and preparation. The President's trip to Cairo and Jerusalem, and the negotiations involved with it, occurred in the full glare of press scrutiny, in two foreign countries, with minimal time for the planning and preparation that precedes the most routine presidential trip abroad, which this most assuredly was not.

The one great similarity was the psychological and diplomatic context. In both cases there was an overwhelming sense of urgency, even desperation. The fourth estate understood, as did the government officials involved: both efforts were long-shot, last-ditch attempts. If they were unsuccessful, the consequences would be unpredictable at best.

Even in this area, there was at least one aspect that changed significantly between the meeting at Camp David and the Cairo-Jerusalem shuttle. Relations between press and White House were frayed and tattered by the summer of 1978; six months later they were even worse.

As one might expect, both the psychological-diplomatic context and the settings of the two events had a profound effect upon the behavior of journalists and government officials.

Since this is not a diplomatic history, there is no need to replay in detail the maneuvering and negotiating tactics that were employed at Camp David. However, it is important for the reader to remember what led up to the highly charged atmosphere that existed in the summer of 1978: President Carter had entered office with the Middle East as one of his most important foreign-policy priorities. He and his principal advisers felt that the time was right for a full-court press toward a comprehensive peace agreement involving Israel and all her Arab neighbors. This included a resolution of the Palestinian problem.

The stalemate that existed in 1977 was inherently unstable, bound to be broken sooner or later by either progress or by war. If there was to be a nuclear confrontation between the superpowers, the Middle East was the most likely place for it. The President understood very well that his leverage at home and abroad would never be greater than during his first year in office, and he was determined to waste no time in using it.

A series of high-level meetings to plan the American approach were held during the first two weeks of the administration. By the middle of February, Secretary of State Cyrus Vance was on his way to the Middle East for consultations. During his first 108 days in office, the President met for lengthy discussions with Prime Minister Rabin of Israel, President Sadat of Egypt, King Hussein of Jordan, Prince Fahd of Saudi Arabia, and President Assad of Syria.

The President and his foreign policy advisers decided in these early meetings that the only existing mechanism for bringing all the parties together was the Geneva Conference, a mechanism established during the Nixon administration, to be chaired jointly by the United States and the Soviet Union.

The Soviets had played an essentially negative role in the region from the beginning, but over the past several years that role had profited them little. Their ejection from Egypt was a severe setback, relegating them to a somewhat secondary role in the diplomacy of the region. They were still in a position to make the achievement of a comprehensive peace extremely difficult, if not impossible, but there were indications that they might be willing to play a more constructive role in return for being given a place at the table.

The challenge to the President and his team was to induce the Soviets to be constructive without adding to their influence in a way that would be detrimental to the United States.

After a series of disappointments and interruptions, including the election of a new Israeli Prime Minister, the President and his advisers believed they had found a way to take at least a small step forward. Following a series of meetings, the Soviet ambassador to Washington presented to the State Department a draft of a joint United States–Soviet statement that could serve as a basis for convening the Geneva Conference.

The statement, which was designed as a listing of agreed principles, contained language that was clearly more moderate than the earlier Soviet positions, and after intense discussions became even more so. On October 1, the President's birthday, it was released to the press in Washington and in Moscow.

Seldom has a President received what turned out to be a more unpleasant birthday surprise. The reaction was immediate, intense, and almost uniformly negative. It was denounced by almost everyone concerned, except Sadat, who saw it as a way to put pressure on Syria to be more reasonable. Within a few days it became clear that the joint statement was a nonstarter.

Whatever the diplomatic merits or shortcomings of the proposal, its handling, particularly in the areas of press and political relations, left much to be desired.

Everyone had underestimated the potential fallout from the news. The press and political operations in the White House had not been brought into the picture until just before the statement was to be released, and we made no serious effort to get a delay so the proper groundwork could be laid.

Many of us were still aching from the resignation of Bert Lance, which had come only a few days before. (The one who had been hurt the most, outside of Bert himself, was the President.)

I remember sitting with Hamilton Jordan late one afternoon

in the immediate aftermath of the Geneva Conference fiasco. We both felt we had done the President a disservice by not arguing more forcefully, much earlier that the fight to keep Bert was lost and that the debilitating controversy had to be ended—for his sake and for Bert's. Now we were forced to admit that we had failed him again. The fact that older and wiser heads had also misjudged the Geneva initiative was no consolation.

Our dejection and disappointment, and that of those who were working full time on the Middle East, were essentially unrelieved for the next month. Then on November 9, Anwar Sadat announced that he was ready to go to Jerusalem and talk peace with Israeli Prime Minister Menachem Begin. A few days later Mr. Begin responded affirmatively. A new day had dawned. Sadat had almost single-handedly created a new structure to replace the Geneva Conference. The efforts of the American government were turned immediately to supporting and encouraging his initiative and to seeking ways to involve other Arab leaders in the process.

It is indicative of the pretentious nature of the media that this potentially momentous event shortly became an excuse for a tacky quarrel between the networks over whose anchorperson had really been responsible for bringing Begin and Sadat together. If we were disappointed in the White House that President Carter never received the Nobel Peace Prize for his efforts, imagine the chagrin in New York that Walters and Cronkite missed out, too.

One indication of our deteriorating relationship with the press, and an early sign that Carter would receive the minimum credit possible no matter what he did, was the wide currency given to the idea that Sadat's move had come out of desperation and disappointment in American diplomacy. Even after Sadat publicly credited a personal letter from President Carter written on October 21 as being the motivation for his offering to go to Jerusalem, the effort to make it appear that the breakthrough had come despite all the hard work by the President and his advisers continued. Nor has the revelation that Sadat personally welcomed the much maligned Geneva initiative, referring to it as a "master stroke," appreciably altered this perception.

Whatever Sadat's motivations, and I suspect they were in part the same as those that drove President Carter—a recognition that the stalemate had to be broken one way or another—he raised the hopes and prospects for peace to their highest level in thirty years with a single stroke.

Unfortunately, within less than a year those high hopes came up hard against the perplexing realities of the region.

It had quickly become apparent that other Arab nations were not prepared to follow Sadat's lead, and that Sadat and Begin by themselves were making little progress. Accordingly, the United States found itself, by the invitation of all concerned, back in the middle of the process before the end of December. And by January of 1978, Sadat had become so frustrated that he sent word to President Carter that he was ready to withdraw from further negotiations with Israel. Visits to Washington by Sadat in February and Begin in March, plus trips to the region by Vance and Mondale, produced little reason for optimism.

In July, the President sent Vance to meet with the Foreign Ministers of Egypt and Israel at Leeds Castle in Great Britain to try to pick up the pieces. The effort was singularly unsuccessful. The meetings degenerated into public acrimony that mirrored, and to some extent exacerbated, the lack of progress.

Shortly after Secretary Vance returned with confirmation that the talks had in fact been as unproductive as the press accounts had led everyone to believe, President Carter made what may have been the most important decision of his presidency.

He would invite Sadat and Begin to Washington for three-way discussions. His goal, kept secret from all except his closest advisers, would be not just to salvage the Sadat initiative, but to bring about peace and diplomatic recognition between Israel and Egypt and to create a framework that would bring the other parties to the conflict, including the Palestinians, into the negotiations.

Secretary Vance was dispatched with letters of invitation to Sadat and Begin. They quickly accepted. On August 8, we announced that a summit on the Middle East would take place beginning the first week in September.

The announcement was actually made while Vance was still in the Middle East. The reason was to forestall leaks from either Jerusalem or Cairo, which would have almost certainly had a spin to them that would have made the other side uncomfortable.

This was the first in a series of actions designed to restrain or preempt leaks and the diplomatic consequences that can result from them. Indeed, the relationship between the White House and the press during the Camp David summit would be dominated by our attempts to prevent the unauthorized or premature disclosure of information.

Holding the summit at Camp David was not a part of the original decision. It could have gone down in history by a variety of other names: Blair House, Jackson Place, Meridian House, Dumbarton Oaks, maybe even the Sheraton-Carlton. But as we looked at alternative sites, it became clear that none suited our purposes nearly so well as the presidential retreat in the Catoctin mountains.

At the top of the list was the question of privacy. Following the abortive conference at Leeds Castle, I had been almost as interested in debriefing State Department spokesman Hodding Carter as in hearing what his boss had to say.

Hodding had been decidedly unhappy about the press operations. He was convinced that the nonstop leaking of comments and positions from the negotiations, primarily for the purpose of making the participants look good back home and pinning the blame for failure on the other parties, had made a situation that was bad enough at the outset virtually impossible.

There was only one solution. Keep the participants away from reporters. And it clearly had to be done physically. Appeals for self-restraint were likely to be about as effective as urging houseflies to avoid sour milk. (Hodding is from Mississippi and readily grasped the analogy between flies and diplomats, as well as the correlation between the press and sour milk; others involved in the decision had to have the analogy explained for them.)

If one is looking for a place to lock up a group of distinguished officials for an extended period of time and deny them easy access to anyone on the outside, it would be hard to find a better one than Camp David.

Although less than two hours from Washington by car, thirty minutes by presidential helicopter, Camp David is about as secluded as a place can be. Perched atop a mountain in the Catoctins, surrounded by a double-fence security perimeter that is patrolled regularly by a special marine detachment, the former

CCC camp has been a haven of peace and solitude for American Presidents since FDR.

The only concession to press coverage is a small fenced path just inside the main gate leading to an area, screened by small evergreens, from which photographers are allowed to watch the presidential helicopter land and take off.

The grudging nature of this bow to the somewhat macabre "body-watch" by the fourth estate is made even more explicit by the understanding that no photos will be used unless something extraordinary happens—presumably the President falling out the door of Marine One, debarking with a starlet on each arm, or the helicopter itself crashing in flames. There is an eminently practical reason for this restriction: most First Ladies do not care to get fixed up for a public appearance every time they arrive or depart Camp David.

The screen of evergreens was planted on orders from President Nixon and a three-sided enclosure was erected for the photographers to stand behind once the helicopter had landed and their photographs had been taken. Rumor has it that Mr. Nixon did not want to have to look at them as he drove by on his way to the presidential cabin—an emotion that every modern President must have shared at one time or another.

The accommodations at Camp David are comfortable but not plush. Mrs. Kennedy reportedly described them as "early Holiday Inn" and refused to spend much time there. But all subsequent Presidents have been indebted to President Nixon for making the facilities even more comfortable and convenient. He had a new lodge constructed that provided a staff dining area, a large informal living room, and two meeting rooms. Two other meeting rooms are available a few steps away in an older building that also houses the pool table.

Everyone who enters or leaves the area passes through a single gate manned by marine guards who routinely record "who" and "when" each time the gate is opened.

All of the necessary services are handled by military personnel. There are no civilian cooks, waiters, maids, or even yardmen to provide tidbits of gossip to enterprising reporters.

Both the distance from Washington and a policy that all those involved in the negotiations must stay at Camp David discouraged a flow of aides and advisers in and out, and made it unlikely that anyone who knew what was happening would be sitting down for a drink and a friendly chat with a journalist.

Telephone calls are handled through a central switchboard, staffed by the Army Signal Corps. Although no calls were monitored during the summit, I suspected that our guests were never quite sure and were thus more inclined to limit telephone conversations with reporters.

A proposal to install eavesdropping devices in the rooms used by our guests was vetoed by the President. I agreed with the decision, but I must confess that my position had more to do with the expectation that word of the eavesdropping would leak than with a refined sense of propriety.

Our hope was that all of this would discourage public negotiations through the press, which could wreck the summit. The chances that the President could achieve his goals were slim as it was. He deserved every bit of an edge that we could provide.

The source of the difficulties we were trying to avoid can be found in two characteristics of journalists and government officials. The press has an incurable tendency to hype any public comment by one side and then race to someone on the other side with the most provocative interpretation possible in hopes of eliciting a response that is as provocative as the question.

Heads of state and government are politicians, first and foremost, and they have an incurable tendency to play to public constituencies at home and abroad.

Even if Prime Minister A realizes that the press is hyping the comments of his counterpart from the other side, he is still in a bind. The people back home are not going to read and hear exactly what was said by his opposite number. They are going to get the juiced-up version.

Perhaps he can get by with explaining that the press accounts were not quite accurate, providing he is sure the fellow on the other side will not cut his legs out from under him by adopting the more provocative version to keep from looking like he has backed down.

He may be able to beg off by saying he wants to see the full text of the remarks, hoping that attention will have shifted by the next day.

He may even get away with the soft answer that turneth away wrath, but he had better not try that too often if he does not want to turn *on* the wrath of the hardliners back home.

One of these or a similar dodge is used, more often than not, to blunt efforts to provoke. But every now and then, particularly as the situation becomes more tense, as fatigue sets in and patience grows thin, Prime Minister A responds in kind. Then both sides become publicly committed to positions that are unreasonable and devoid of nuance, and the task of reconciliation becomes even more difficult.

Neither press nor public officials are inherently evil. But when mixed together under certain circumstances, the combination can constitute a clear and present danger to world peace and the welfare of the Republic.

A relatively harmless but troublesome example of exactly the sort of thing we were trying to prevent began on August 30 with a report that Carter was considering the stationing of American troops in the Middle East to guarantee a peace agreement.

It all started with a shouted question as the President was boarding Air Force One to return from his vacation in Wyoming. (I have little doubt that World War III, if and when it comes, will be triggered by some American President's partially understood response to a half-heard, shouted question as he is boarding an airplane.)

The wire services immediately reported that the President had suggested that he was keeping that option open for discussion at Camp David. The suggestion was all in their heads. The pool report quote was "He'd be reluctant to do it. We'll just have to wait and see."

CBS and NBC played it straight and well down in their shows, but ABC—whose White House correspondent, Sam Donaldson, had shouted the original question—hyped the story to a fare-thee-well. Mr. Donaldson changed the President's comment, which definitely was a negative response, to a report that Carter had "confirmed in effect" that he might offer U.S. forces. He then opined that the fact that such ideas were even being considered was proof of how grim the administration believed the future would be if the summit failed.

This is an example of a story that was virtually created from whole cloth because one reporter came up with a provocative question and then led the way in distorting the answer.

And in this case the reporting had reverberations. Prime Minister Begin immediately and publicly rejected an idea that was never proposed. The next night, Thursday, August 31, ABC was able to parlay the Wyoming airport gambit into a two-day story. The network led its evening news show with a two-minute report of Begin's rejection and a report by Ted Koppel at the State Department informing viewers that *Begin was responding to a trial balloon, leaked from the White House!*

This sort of thing has some of the qualities of a reporter torching a warehouse, phoning in the alarm, and then filing a story on the evils of arson after the east wall falls on a fire engine.

Appropriately, we on that very day announced that I would be the sole spokesman for the summit. This was an effort to reduce the chances of just this sort of controversy. It was a specific reaction to the problems that had developed at Leeds Castle when all three governments briefed reporters in one fashion or another almost every day.

The idea did not come from me but from Secretary Vance. When the President told me about it, I was somewhat hesitant about the reaction of my Egyptian and Israeli counterparts. Had I been in their position, the idea of turning over my briefing responsibilities to the spokesman of a foreign government would have provoked an extremely negative reaction.

As it turned out there was initial resistance on both sides. Their concerns, as might have been expected, focused primarily on the handling of their own reporters.

Dan Patir, the Israeli spokesman, was not at all sure that I could handle the Israeli press, which he accurately described as "even more aggressive and sensationalist than the Americans."

The Egyptians, who were in a better position to influence what was reported domestically, were less concerned, as long as they were allowed some informal channels to get the official line out to their journalists.

Nevertheless, neither government raised serious objections to the idea of a single American briefer. I was surprised, to say the least.

In retrospect, I think we may have been surprised because we did not, perhaps could not, understand how badly the other two governments wanted peace. We saw the issues as being humanitarian, but in theoretical terms, as a problem affecting long-term stability and U.S. interests in the region. Their friends and families had been fighting and dying there for the past thirty years. If this summit failed, their sons and grandsons might very well be fighting and dying for the next three decades. We also may have underestimated the relief they felt at having the press off their backs for a few days at least.

As it turned out, both the Egyptians and the Israelis maintained fairly regular contact with their journalists. Although this was a violation of the rules that had been established, we chose not to make an issue of it because the information provided was always limited. Nor was there any evidence that these "informal" channels were being used in a way that would jeopardize the undertakings.

The only problem that resulted was a certain amount of complaining from American reporters that their Egyptian and Israeli counterparts were getting "background briefings" from inside the camp. To alleviate their concerns, I began staying around the press center after my formal briefings to chat with American reporters on a not-for-attribution basis. That, plus the restraint shown by the Israeli and Egyptian briefers, kept the issues from becoming serious.

Once we knew who the briefer would be, the next question was where to do the briefing. Camp David itself was out. There were no adequate facilities. Even if there had been, the last thing we wanted was several hundred reporters roaming around the area.

The President felt even more strongly about this than I did. Several weeks before the summit began, I presented to him a memo describing my plans to provide photo opportunities inside the camp each day. My theory was that this would relieve some of the pressure, at least from the networks. He rejected the idea. I could not budge him.

As it turned out, one of the reasons for his stand was a letter from Mamie Eisenhower that had arrived on his desk at about the same time as my memo. She expressed her pride that the camp named for her grandson was again to be the site of an effort to bring peace to the world, and she wished the President the best of luck. However, she also said that she hoped the privacy of Camp David would be preserved. She was concerned that once it was breached by herds of reporters and photographers, it would never be private again. President Carter agreed with her completely, and that was that.

The nearest possible location for a press center and briefing room was the small Maryland town of Thurmont, about thirty minutes down the mountain from Camp David. But Thurmont, which to its credit had remained largely unaffected by its proximity to the presidential retreat, could not provide lodging for all the reporters who would cover the summit.

What we needed was adequate space under one roof for a filing center, staff offices, and a briefing room. A White House advance and communications team was dispatched to see what could be arranged. After several days of searching the advancemen recommended that we lease the Thurmont American Legion hall.

The logistic and communications preparations for the press were, as is often the case, almost as complicated and expensive as those for the participants. At the top of the mountain were three principal actors, Carter, Begin, and Sadat, plus some two dozen aides and advisers. Arrayed about the foot of the mountain were as many as fifteen hundred press personnel. The State Department credentialed more than eleven hundred newspeople—in addition to several hundred who already held White House press passes.

To enable the press to report the scanty information available, Ma Bell set up portable microwave units to handle the surge in telephone traffic, which would otherwise have completely swamped the circuits available in the small town. Eighteen teletype machines and two hundred special telephone lines were installed. The telephone lines included one direct line to Cairo for the Egyptian press and fourteen phones at the foot of a tree near the small wooden CAMP DAVID sign just outside the main gate.

That small sign, which stands against a background of green trees and bushes, became a familiar sight to millions of Americans over the next several days and a bone of contention between the White House Press Office and the networks.

With no access to any part of Camp David and a desperate need to show their viewers that they were indeed on the scene, the network anchors and correspondents quickly identified the sign as absolutely the only place to do their stand-ups for morning and evening news broadcasts.

At first, free access to that all-important spot was allowed, but the coming and going of vans and limousines filled with anchors, retainers, correspondents, and technicians soon created a miniature Santa Monica Freeway. Despite anguished protests from the networks, an outer perimeter was established several hundred yards away from where the camp road branched off Manahan Road. Representatives of the Secret Service and the White House Press Office were stationed there to escort network crews to the sign during prearranged hours of the day.

Problems for the nets did not end with access to the sign, however. They still had to find a way to get a live signal from Camp David to the network itself.

CBS tried a helicopter with a trailing antenna. Unfortunately, the *whump-whump* of the chopper proved to be plainly audible and somewhat distracting in the meeting rooms at Camp David. After private appeals to CBS failed to alleviate the problem, a request was made to the Federal Aviation Administration to extend the area over Camp David from which aircraft were prohibited. Fortunately, at about the same time, CBS discovered that their chopper-borne antenna produced less than ideal pictures, and peace and quiet were restored to the summit conferees.

ABC tried a helium-filled balloon, with an equal lack of success. Not only was the signal poor, but there was difficulty in keeping it aloft. This resulted in part from the fact that some among the local citizenry considered it great sport to take long-distance potshots at the balloon with their deer rifles.

Whether they were encouraged in this by the two competing networks has never been established. I personally had nothing to do with it and was filled with regret upon learning of the riddled ABC balloon.

Since the President had vetoed my idea of allowing the press into Camp David for photo sessions, White House Press Office photos were the only other pictures available to the networks or the papers and magazines. We tried mightily to provide a selection from which they chose every day.

A darkroom was set up at Camp David for black and white photos. Since color development and printing could not be done there, and the nets did not want to use black and white, color film was flown by helicopter to the Navy lab in Anacostia, about forty minutes away, and back to Camp David for selection and distribution.

Each day, prior to release, the pictures to be distributed were first presented to the Egyptian and Israeli press spokesmen for their approval. It simply would not do to release a set of pictures that showed more of Begin than Sadat, or that placed one or the other in a more favorable perspective. You could not have Carter and Sadat smiling while Begin looked dour, or vice versa.

This clearing of photos turned out to be even more complicated than we had expected, because Osama el-Baz, the Egyptian spokesman, became a key negotiator. He spent more time with President Carter than Sadat and Begin combined, and was thus one of the hardest people at the conference to reach on short notice. How could I explain to the nets that their pictures for that day were late because Osama was sitting around with Carter chatting about troop withdrawals, oil rights, the status of Jerusalem, and other less urgent matters?

After President Sadat left Camp David on the second day for a private tour of the countryside without notifying the press, all three networks maintained a permanent stakeout with correspondent, camera crew, and automobile at the Manahan Road gate.

Such stakeouts are seldom productive and often boring as well as uncomfortable for the crews assigned to them. Usually, card games and liar's poker keep them marginally sane. In this case, Jim Duffy, a CBS cameraman, came up with a more productive and less risky endeavor. He bought a woodburning set and spent his time producing souvenir press tags by burning "Camp David Summit—Sept. 1978" into small pieces of wood. His enterprise became so successful among the reporters assembled at Thurmont that Secret Service and White House press staffers began to watch for the "Duffy press passes" as well as the official credentials when clearing reporters into restricted areas.

The briefing room and filing center were situated in a large ballroom-gymnasium on the second floor of the American Legion hall. Working space for the White House Press Office was located downstairs. While the filing center upstairs was often quiet and almost deserted, the staff area was in constant turmoil. There were no private offices, only curtained partitions obtained from the White House Communications Agency. At times conversation became almost impossible over the ringing, rumbling clatter of phones, typewriters, and copying machines.

In the thirteen days of the summit, the press office typed, duplicated, and distributed more than one hundred thousand legal-size pages of transcripts, schedules, notices, and statements—the sum total of which contained about five paragraphs of good hard news.

Between the staff offices and the briefing room was the American Legion bar. It opened early and stayed open late. With its commanding view of the whole disorderly process, it became a favorite vantage point for the natives of Thurmont. The fifty-cent drinks made it equally popular with the press and staff.

This unique opportunity for an entire small town to watch the White House Press Office and the major part of the international press corps at work must have had a lasting impact. It is my suspicion that a poll of the citizens of Thurmont would find that even to this day they are less inclined to trust a statement emanating from the White House or a report from a major news organization than any other group of people on the face of the earth.

Under the mutually agreed, but never written out, rules for the briefing, I was to describe the meetings that had taken place since the last briefing and provide a little "color" on the nonsubstantive activities of the participants—"Prime Minister Begin played chess with Dr. Brzezinski last night," "President Sadat went for a stroll yesterday afternoon and ran into Mrs. Begin and Mrs. Carter, who were touring the premises in a golf cart," and so forth. I was to check even these headline-grabbing comments with Dan Patir and Osama el-Baz to avoid any possibility of a misunderstanding.

We were all aware that if the summit lasted more than a few days, I would be forced to provide some general characterization of the tone of and perhaps the amount of progress made in the talks. The goal was to avoid any step-by-step, blow-by-blow analysis, to resist the pressure for daily temperature taking, and it was hoped, with only one briefer, to keep conflicts between the parties out of the news. I had been at the job long enough by then to know that avoiding conflict, or at least the appearance of conflict, between statements was not a sure thing even if only one person was speaking.

Certainly, I was never to speak for the Egyptian or Israeli government. Any question as to the positions of either party on the issues under discussion simply could not be answered.

CAMP DAVID EVE

Between the announcement of and the convening of the summit, President Carter left on a vacation visit to Idaho and Wyoming. During that trip I reached what was probably my low point of the entire administration. We were dropping in the polls. Our relations with the press were equally discouraging. I even gave an interview to a local reporter who came away convinced that I was so discouraged that I was thinking of resigning.

I do not think this period of despondency—that is the best word I can think of to describe it; if it was not clinical, it was damn close—was noticed by my staff or others in the White House. I could tell that my wife, Nan, knew something was wrong, but, as is her habit, she did not pry or even raise the subject unless I did.

Even the press coverage of the President's vacation trip was somewhat negative, which only added to my sense of discouragement and futility. I remember thinking that even a jackass as press secretary ought to be able to get a President decent coverage out of a fishing trip.

During the trip, I had several long conversations with reporters, usually over a few drinks on both sides. I particularly remember talking with Muriel Dobbin of the *Baltimore Sun*. She tried to convince me that my strong personal reaction to the negativism in the press was hurting my effectiveness.

I responded that I had every right to be discouraged and angry. The press, I said, was irresponsible and occasionally downright nasty. If she wanted to do some good she ought to be talking to her colleagues about their attitude and behavior instead of counseling me.

I am sure she left thinking her time had been wasted because I never gave any indication that I saw merit in what she had to say. But after returning to Washington, I concluded that she was right.

I can still remember the exact moment when it dawned on me. We had gotten back to Washington on Wednesday, August 30, 1978. Two days later on a Friday night I was reading myself to sleep, as usual. I generally had little trouble falling asleep as long as I had something to read, usually history, to help get my mind off the events of the day. That particular day had not been especially eventful or hectic, which was perhaps the reason I found my mind wandering back to the vacation trip and Muriel's attempt to talk some sense into my head. Whatever criticisms could be leveled at the press, my first concern had to be how I was doing my job, and I clearly had to maintain some degree of detachment if I was going to survive, much less do it properly.

There was nothing very precise about my decision. It was mostly a determination to take a step back, to stop agonizing over things I could do nothing about. The White House press corps, I decided, was what it was, and I was not likely to change it. I had to resign myself to dealing with the institution as it existed.

From that day forward, when the pressures and irritations began to build, I simply looked for a day that could be expected to be routine and spent the morning at home. I was only fifteen minutes from the White House if I had to get there in a hurry, but those mornings away gave me a chance to clear my mind and collect my wits. For the most part, I spent them reading, history again, but absolutely nothing later than the nineteenth century. From early spring through the fall, there was our rose garden to work in. I could take out my frustrations on aphids and black spot instead of ABC and the *Boston Globe*. (By the end of the administration, the rose garden was much improved. I wish I could say the same for the President's image. On the other hand, I never tried spraying the press room once a week and after every rain shower with captan and Malathion.)

I was right in deciding not to let things get to me so badly, but I was wrong though in thinking, as I did at the time, that a better attitude on my part would produce a better attitude toward the President on the part of the press. It did not.

At best, my more philosophical approach may have kept me from becoming so ineffective that I could not function at all. With the summit coming up, my change in attitude could not have come at a more propitious time. There is no doubt that had I entered that period in the same mental state I was in when we left for the Far West, press relations at Camp David would have been a disaster.

The few days after the end of the vacation were also a propitious time for me to make a change in my attitude and approach to the job. For that period, the principal story was the upcoming summit. We had the initiative and since nothing had yet happened, there was little to argue with the press about. There was also a certain relief in focusing on a single priority. Usually, the press office and the press corps are juggling three or four potentially explosive stories each day.

Essentially, we were marking time. The air was filled with anticipation rather than tension and acrimony. And there was also hope, a sentiment that was shared by many of those covering the White House. They understood the stakes and the risks as well as we did. A few even found the chance to slip into my office to offer a handshake and a half-embarrassed "Good luck."

Walter Cronkite best summed up the mood and feel of that time on the evening before Sadat and Begin were to arrive at Camp David: "The best thing the negotiators have going for them is that there is so much to lose if the summit is a failure."

The public positions put forward by the parties had become reasonably accurate reflections of their actual postures. Sadat was inclined to take the long view. He saw time as being on his side, and he retained the option of returning to the Arab fold if the effort was a failure.

Begin was worried, as most Israeli premiers have been, about pressure from the United States—his only real ally. He had been forced to expend more effort than his predecessors to keep his own country and the American Jewish community united behind him, and he had deep emotional and security concerns about the yielding of occupied territory, which he knew would be necessary to gain peace.

Carter was not just posturing when he warned of the disastrous consequences of failure. But he knew, perhaps better than either Sadat or Begin, how far each would need to move to make an agreement possible, and he hoped that constant public reminders of what was at stake would pressure both to be more flexible.

The first sour note in the area of press relations was struck shortly after the summit began. On Wednesday, September 6, I announced that the press would be invited to a performance of the Marine Silent Drill Team to be held at Camp David the next evening. Their behavior at that event is one of the more unpleasant memories from my four years at the White House.

Since space was limited, we had to prohibit some of the families of marine and Navy personnel on the Camp David staff from attending to make room for the press.

Because we knew they would feel compelled to try to snag some of the participants in the talks for interviews, we took special pains to keep the two groups apart. We should have recognized that being so close to the principals but unable to get to them would be too much for the press to bear.

There were numerous complaints that steps taken to keep them away from the participants were excessive, even as several reporters made every effort to evade the precautions. A few even tried to hide in the network technical trailers so they could jump out and grab someone when the participants came by.

There was also the usual grumbling from photographers about not being in a position to get all the shots they wanted. Some of the cursing and shouting from the photogs was loud enough to distract attention from the ceremony. The crowning blow came with the playing of the national anthem. The press corps, with a few exceptions, refused to stand.

I could not believe my eyes. American reporters, the most privileged journalists on the face of the earth and in the history of the world, expressing their pique about logistic arrangements through disrespect to the flag. The "visual" was dramatic: three hundred Americans, Israelis, and Egyptians standing silently as the color guard presented arms and the marine band boomed the national anthem into the night, while a few dozen American reporters sat sullenly, complaining so loudly that everyone in attendance could hear them.

My wife was so angry that she had tears in her eyes when I saw her a few minutes later. She and our eleven-year-old daughter, and a few press office staffers, had been seated in the press section. When they rose for the presentation of the colors and the national anthem, a few reporters had cursed and shouted at them to sit down.

After the ceremony I complained to several correspondents about their behavior. Most of them were unable to remember the incident or claimed to have been among the few who did stand. Among those who heard my angry reaction were the two White House correspondents from *Newsweek*. The next week there was a story on the complaints of the press about the way they had been treated at the ceremony. In typical *Newsweek* fashion, the refusal to stand for the flag and the national anthem was not mentioned.

So far as I have been able to tell, not one word was ever written about this incident anywhere—a stark contrast to what seemed to us to be the eagerness to report any real or imagined breach of protocol by White House staffers, particularly if they happened to have been born in Georgia. It is worth noting only because it illustrates one of the characteristics of press behavior that was the most irritating to those of us on the other side: a double standard for judging what is acceptable behavior, and by extension what is newsworthy. It would crop up again and again during the months to come.

On Saturday the ninth, I announced that President Carter would take President Sadat and Prime Minister Begin to tour the Gettysburg battlefield on Sunday. The announcement was made "for guidance only," which means that the press can use the information for planning purposes but cannot report it. This term of art is often used when a President wishes to go somewhere without a public announcement.

Generally, the press respects the ground rules because there is a security consideration. The chances of a successful attack on a President are greatly reduced if there is no advance notice to a potential assassin. Security problems are further reduced because crowds are smaller with no advance notice. In this case, we had two Presidents and a Prime Minister to worry about, so everyone was more nervous than usual.

The press corps also recognizes that fewer security problems and smaller crowds usually mean better access for them, and they know that the President can always go without telling them at all.

As usual, however, there was squabbling about any attempt to prohibit the reporters from reporting everything they knew. Part of the squabbling is intended as a deterrent, to make the press secretary's life uncomfortable enough to minimize the use of such restraints. Part stems from the fear that someone else will violate the ground rules and gain a competitive advantage—this concern is particularly keen among the wire services, which measure success in being only a few minutes ahead of the competition on almost any bit of news.

The trip to Gettysburg arose partially out of a comment by Prime Minister Begin that he would like to visit the battlefield. However, the President's invitation was motivated by more than courtesy and a desire to escape the confines of Camp David.

Earlier in the administration, the President had visited both Gettysburg and Sharpsburg (or Antietam, if your great-granddaddy fought on the wrong side), accompanied by Shelby Foote, author of perhaps the finest history of the Civil War ever written. As a southerner and as a President with the power to send men to fight and die, he had been moved and impressed by what he saw.

The Civil War (or War Between the States, if your family was on the right side) provides for southerners a perspective that differs from that of most Americans. Tales of glory and valor are forever entwined with bitter memories of defeat, humiliation, and terrible loss. In the South, one fourth of all white males of military age were killed or wounded in less than four years. The South of the President's childhood still suffered in substance and spirit from that loss, and even on that Sunday morning 115 years later, recovery was not yet complete.

But that bloodiest of American wars also spoke to the possibility of reconciliation, of the ability of each side to grant to the other the sincerity of the convictions for which it fought and to honor the sacrifices made. It spoke to the hope that death and destruction might give rise, not to more violence and hate, but to a determination "to avoid the useless sacrifice . . . that must have attended the continuance of this contest."

President Carter understood, in a way that another President might not, the experience of Arab and Israeli. I thought at the time that perhaps he hoped, with that visit to the place where fifty thousand young men had fallen, to let Sadat and Begin know that he understood and to remind them of what was at stake.

What effect, if any, the visit had on President Sadat or Prime Minister Begin I do not know. If either spoke privately to the President about it, he has never recounted the conversation. But looking back, another thought occurs to me. Perhaps it was President Carter who benefited most from the impact of the visit. He was keenly aware, as he said in an interview shortly before the summit began, that what was at stake was peace or war not just for Israel and Egypt, but perhaps for the United States as well. In the week following that trip to Gettysburg, there would be times of discouragement and intense frustration, when the temptation to give up would arise. The Civil War, even more than most wars, had been a result of the failure of politics and the shortsightedness of politicians. Maybe it was also a good thing for Jimmy Carter to be reminded of what he understood about war and the consequences of failure.

It was on Monday the eleventh, while the Camp David talks were reaching a critical stage, that syndicated columnist Jack Anderson informed the nation that Hamilton Jordan and Charles Kirbo, the President's longtime friend, were involved in an effort to get the Justice Department to back away from attempts to extradite fugitive financier and former Nixon confidant Robert Vesco.

Anderson had called me about the story on Saturday. After checking with Hamilton, I denied that anything improper had occurred and begged Anderson for the time I needed to prove to him with files and phone logs that no one had ever asked Hamilton to take any role in a matter that the Justice Department was pursuing aggressively. He refused and went ahead with a column and a piece on ABC's *Good Morning America*.

Hamilton and I were concerned enough to fly down to Washington on Sunday for a meeting on the subject. We learned that the *Washington Post* had refused to run the column unless it was substantially altered, and that Anderson had complied with requests from Executive Editor Ben Bradlee to greatly soften the allegations.

This prompted an attempt by us to get Anderson and/or his syndicate to request that other papers hold the column until the rewritten version could be gotten to them. The request was refused.

The charges were proven to be without foundation, but only after a grand jury investigation and a great deal of unfavorable publicity.

It turned out that the one piece of hard evidence Anderson had to support his contentions was a copy of a letter that allegedly had been written to Vesco by Hamilton on White House stationery. When we finally saw the letter we knew it was an obvious forgery. The format and the letterhead were totally unlike any that ever came out of our, or any other, administration.

Anderson was finally forced to admit that it was a fake. But he stuck by his story anyway, claiming the letter was a "reconstruction" of an actual letter that had somehow been misplaced.

Anderson's behavior in this instance destroyed what little confidence I had left in his integrity. It also foreshadowed an even more scandalous episode during the hostage crisis.

Since I will return to the subject of Jack Anderson several times before this book is finished, my point of view needs to be established right at the start.

In the course of my four years in the White House, I came to the conclusion that Jack Anderson was dangerously unreliable. In the three years since, I have discovered that this opinion is shared by a large number of the more respected journalists in Washington. However, because of their reluctance to criticize another member of the fourth estate, those opinions are not known by millions of Americans who read Anderson's columns in hundreds of newspapers.

That is not proper. If the press feels there is reason to doubt the integrity of a public official, they will make sure that warning is conveyed to their readers and viewers. Isn't there a similar obligation with regard to someone with as much power and influence on public policy as Anderson?

* * *

On the same day we were dealing with the false Anderson story, ABC once again raised the issue of stationing American troops in the Middle East, despite my strong denial that this was under consideration. After saying that Carter was now "setting out his own proposals," which I had confirmed to him on deep background that afternoon, Sam Donaldson added, ". . . perhaps offering the use of U.S. forces—we don't know."

That made four separate stories out of this nonproposal in less than two weeks. In addition to the original two, the ever resourceful Mr. Donaldson had used a visit to Camp David by Defense Secretary Harold Brown three days earlier to report that I had denied that his visit had to do with considerations of stationing troops in the Middle East.

This dogged persistence, this almost fanatical determination never to admit error, is one of the least endearing and most counterproductive characteristics of the fourth estate. It is by no means confined to Mr. Donaldson or to television reporting. It does vary among individual reporters and news organizations, but it is almost always there in some degree.

The original mistake may have been justifiable or at least understandable. The hardheaded determination to persist in and compound error is virtually without parallel except in the Supreme Soviet or a disturbed adolescent.

When I lit into Donaldson the day after the fourth story, in terms much more heated and colorful than those above, he brushed it off with humor, as he often did when I came at him with my hackles up.

"Ah, young man," he said, "you say no troops, but mark my words, there will be American troops there before we're done." A prediction he pointed to with feigned pride four years later when President Reagan dispatched marines to Lebanon. I had to laugh, as I had four years prior, despite my irritation.

Only four days later, the focus of press interest returned to the question of a bad personal relationship between Sadat and Begin. There was a rumor that Sadat had threatened to break off the summit and return to Egypt. This rumor was true, although I did not know it at the time. When asked if there had been such a crisis last night, I said, "No!" By that afternoon I had checked with the

President and he confirmed the rumor. Although my statement at the briefing had not been intentionally deceptive, it was, nevertheless, completely false.

I was concerned, but not excessively so. I believed there was an obligation to correct the record, but I feared that what would amount to an announcement from the conference spokesman that Sadat had threatened to go home would be both improper and not very helpful. I decided to wait until the conference was over. As it turned out, President Sadat took care of the matter himself in an interview with Walter Cronkite on the day after the summit ended.

That situation is one of many that go to the heart of the question of whether it is possible for a press secretary to know too much. In general, I think the answer is no. If something needs to be kept confidential, my experience has been that a spokesman can usually do a better job if he knows what he is trying to protect. This can usually be accomplished with a dodge or nonanswer that stops short of a flat untruth. Had I known about the Sadat incident before I got the first question, I could simply have said, "You will have to check with President Sadat on that," or "The last time I checked, he was still here and had no plans to leave until the conference is over," or words to that effect.

Occasionally, there are cases where the information to be protected is so sensitive, and the likelihood that anything other than a straight denial will be read as a confirmation so strong, the only alternative may be to lie. If the matter is that important, it is all the more reason for the spokesman to know exactly what is to be protected so he can do an effective job of constructing and presenting a cover story. I was to face such a situation almost two years later during the Iran crisis.

Anyway, by the end of the first week the general question of the relationship between Sadat and Begin had become a regular topic at my briefings, spurred by the fact, obvious from the schedule of meetings we posted each day, that the two had not met personally since the second day.

I had tried for several days to avoid the issue without either implying a confirmation or flatly saying something that was not true. In looking back over my earlier briefings, I felt an obligation to give the press at least a hint that they might be on the right track. I also felt that since we were close to the end of the conference, anything short of a direct confirmation would not jeopardize the outcome.

During the thirty-minute briefing on Friday of the second week—the same briefing where Sadat's threat to leave arose—there were thirteen questions on the Sadat-Begin relationship.

The first thing I had to do was to find a way to declare my earlier comments "inoperative" without being explicit or quotable.

The most obvious tactic was simply to refuse to deny the first negative characterization of the relationship that came up. When I was asked whether "the relations between the two [Sadat and Begin] are so poor that those two men cannot sit down together," I evaded but did not deny.

The second method was humor, perhaps the most effective tool in any spokesman's kit. It can relieve tension, disrupt the rhythm of an aggressive line of questioning, and, as in this case, convey serious information to the astute reporter in a manner that is almost impossible to quote in a serious story.

Helen Thomas, of UPI, informed me, rather emphatically and early in the briefing, that my usual assertion—the lack of meetings between the two was merely a part of the normal flow of things, and of no particular significance—would not sell anymore. I responded that in that case I would like to try to sell them "a new set of pots and pans" and asking whether they might be willing "to buy some aluminum siding" instead—a clear indication that what I had said in the past and was about to say now should be taken with a grain of salt.

When the reporters realized that I was not going to flatly deny the rumors about bad blood, they pressed hard for a usable quote. I managed to avoid giving them one. Although I doubt there was an experienced newsperson in the room who had any question about the truth of the rumors by the time the briefing was over, only Judy Woodruff of NBC managed to get on the air with a reference to the fact that I had "sidestepped reports of serious animosity between Sadat and Begin." The print reporters made only brief references to the matter, well down in their stories.

The reaction of the reporters after the conference was over—when it became clear to everyone that the personal relations had been awful and that Sadat had indeed threatened to leave on Thursday night—was of particular interest to me, primarily because there was none. I expected to take a fair amount of heat and abuse for my not always too skillful attempts to mislead them, but it never came.

Looking back on it now, the journalists involved cite a variety of reasons why I got off the hook so easily. The one most frequently mentioned is that the summit was a success. There was an air of good feeling and everyone was concentrating in a positive way on how the President had pulled it off, rather than on bitter postmortems of a gamble that failed.

Others emphasize that my deception did not lead anyone to file an erroneous story. The stories that mentioned the Sadat threat merely quoted my denial and let it go at that. In fact, as one journalist pointed out, if I had confirmed the Sadat threat, they would have had extremely pessimistic stories in Saturday's papers—the day before the conference ended as a roaring success. (As I was to learn six months later, at the end of the President's trip to Jerusalem and Cairo, reporters who feel they have been misled *and* who end up with egg on their faces are not inclined to be charitable.)

Finally, a few who say they took note of my transgressions at the time also say they decided not to make an issue of them because they understood and sympathized with my reasons for wanting to downplay such stories. They were, after all, also in favor of peace in the Middle East. Furthermore, they judged my motives as having been acceptable in that the deception had not been designed to improperly benefit the President or the administration, even if they could not officially approve of my methods.

Sunday, September 17, 1978, was one of those days you know you will always remember without having to look at a diary or check your notes. It was the thirteenth day at Camp David. By midmorning it seemed clear that we had achieved a result far beyond our expectations. Not only would there be an agreement on a framework for peace between Israel and Egypt, there would also be an agreement on a framework for continued negotiations toward a comprehensive peace in the region. With the conversion of this framework into an actual treaty of peace, the state of war between Israel and her largest and most powerful Arab neighbor would end for the first time since the creation of Israel.

There was little time for rejoicing, however. Of necessity, little planning had been done for the public ceremonies that would end the summit. Since we had not known whether the summit would end in success or failure or something in between, or even when it would end, only the most general preparations had been possible. Even on Friday, when it became clear that the summit would officially end on Sunday, we could not predict whether that conclusion would come in time for a public announcement that day or whether it would be necessary to wait until Monday. Most of us thought that it would be unlikely to end in time for a Sunday announcement. But we also agreed that we should make every effort to schedule an announcement on Sunday, since reports of the final agreements would almost surely leak overnight, probably in a dangerously distorted form.

There was little doubt in anyone's mind that both the Egyptians and the Israelis would face difficulty in selling the agreement to their respective hardline constituencies. And each delegation would begin as soon as possible to put the best possible face on the concessions each had made. The problem was, of course, that every time Begin attempted to minimize Israeli concessions and emphasize Egyptian concessions he made Sadat's job more difficult, and vice versa. Furthermore, there was still serious negotiating to be done if the frameworks agreed to at Camp David were to be translated into real treaties and agreements, if troops were to be withdrawn, ambassadors exchanged, and borders opened. Distorted and self-serving leaks about the contents of the initial agreements could get these important follow-up negotiations off to a bad start from which they might never recover. We could not prevent this posturing from taking place, but we had to make sure that the first presentation was as accurate and balanced as possible.

With the assurance that success exceeding our most optimistic expectations was only an hour or two away, I called Hodding Carter, the State Department spokesman, and several members of my staff up to Camp David early on Sunday morning. I desperately needed their help and advice in planning and executing an appropriate ceremony in the limited amount of time available to us. They arrived by noon, and we met on the patio at Laurel Lodge, the large, central gathering place for staff and visitors. All other meeting rooms were occupied by negotiators putting the final touches on the agreements.

The weather seemed to have been especially ordered to suit the occasion. The seasons had changed atop the Catoctin mountains during the thirteen days of the summit. Summer was gone and those clear crisp days of early fall were upon us. We sat in shirt sleeves overlooking the peaceful valleys of northwest Maryland and quickly agreed on the essentials of an announcement plan.

There should be a signing ceremony featuring Sadat, Begin, and Carter, in Washington, preferably at the White House. The networks would surely want to carry that ceremony live, and we would need to take into account the time they needed to make the technical arrangements to do so.

Although there was little chance that the documents themselves could be made available to the press on Sunday, we would need some sort of background briefing to supplement whatever comments might be made by the principals at the ceremony. Preferably, the briefing would come after the ceremony, but that would depend on press deadlines and the timing of the announcement. To save time, that briefing would also need to take place in Washington, and the most likely site was the auditorium of the Old Executive Office Building. That auditorium, commonly known as 450 EOB, was virtually next door to the White House and would seat 250 reporters. The EPS guards and the White House Press Office staff were familiar with procedures for clearing the press into the building on short notice.

The press at the American Legion hall in Thurmont would need to be notified of the Washington schedule in time to make the one-and-a-half- to two-hour drive. A ceremony and briefing in Washington with all the press still in Thurmont would have been less than satisfactory from our point of view and theirs.

Two of the national newsmagazines were a special problem. *U.S. News and World Report* has the earliest deadline and had already gone to press. But *Time* and *Newsweek* were still holding their presses on Sunday, hoping to get the conclusion of the summit in the edition that would hit the streets on Monday or Tuesday. If they did not, the ending of the summit would be old news by the time their next editions came out a week later. It was also in our interest to have the triumphful conclusion covered in the current editions. By the next week, the glory and exultation of the moment would almost certainly be tarnished by the inevitable second-guessers and analyzers of the many problems still to be faced.

In such situations it is common practice for the White House press secretary to give informal and off-the-record guidance to news executives to help them plan their coverage and production schedules. On Saturday I had been largely noncommittal, since there was no way of knowing whether there would be an announcement of the results of the summit before Tuesday morning. They decided to take the chance and hold their presses until Sunday. By Sunday at noon, it seemed clear that we would have an announcement by late that afternoon, and I advised them to keep holding. These telephone conversations with the newsmagazines were taking place simultaneously with our planning sessions on the patio at Laurel. Both were interrupted and placed in limbo when Hamilton Jordan stepped onto the patio, motioned me aside, and said the President wanted to see me right away in his cabin.

As we walked the few hundred yards to Aspen Lodge, Hamilton explained that the negotiations had hit a snag over the status of Jerusalem. The successful conclusion, which had been close enough to smell, was now in jeopardy.

The President was in shirt sleeves when he greeted us in the large living room at Aspen. His eyes were slightly red from lack of sleep, and the traces of fatigue and tension were visible in his face. His attitude was a mixture of concern and determination. If there had been a moment of near despair when the potentially fatal snag had developed, he was past it now.

He took only a few minutes to outline the problem and to tell us that he had what he hoped was a solution. He would personally present his plan to Begin and Sadat in less than fifteen minutes. If it worked, we could move ahead as planned. What to do if it did not was what he wanted to talk about. His inclination, as it had been for several days, was to present frankly to the American people and the world a report on the summit, including his explanation of why it had failed. There was no time to reach a definite conclusion before the crucial final meeting, and he would want further discussions with his foreign policy advisers before taking such a dramatic and inevitably controversial step. In the meantime, he wanted to make sure I did nothing that would in any way foreclose that option, and he wanted us to be thinking seriously about our views of the idea. He also knew that I was up to my ears in preparation for the conclusion of the summit, and although he was as usual unconcerned with the details involved, he wanted to let me know of the last-minute hitch so I would not get myself in an embarrassing position with the press.

I raced back to Laurel to tell my colleagues to put everything on hold. A few minutes later when I returned to Aspen, Hamilton was standing on the terrace at the rear of the President's cabin. We could see through the windows that the President was deep in conversation with Osama el-Baz and Aharon Barak, the principal draftsmen for Sadat and Begin respectively. They were working to refine language that had already been agreed upon to resolve the sticking point with regard to Jerusalem. The crisis was already over, but we did not know it.

Finally the President saw us pacing up and down on the terrace, realized our state of mind by our downcast expressions, and gave us a thumbs-up signal. It was done—or almost. Another problem arose a few minutes later over language referring to the Knesset vote on removing the Israeli settlements from the Sinai but was quickly resolved. Hamilton and I clasped hands and slapped each other on the back—rather ridiculous gestures, since neither of us had done anything to be congratulated for. But we both felt the need to congratulate someone, and there was no one else around at the moment.

There was no time for much else in the way of celebrating. Agreement was quickly reached on a schedule for briefing the press and a ceremony to announce the success. I then had thirty minutes to give the appropriate instructions to the press staff in Thurmont and in Washington and get my bags packed to catch the Vice-President's helicopter down to Washington.

Given the hurried nature of arrangements, the events of the rest of the day were a surprising success. The briefing came off with only minor hitches. The ceremony was truly moving, even to some of the more cynical members of the fourth estate.

The only sour note was the reaction of some of the executives at *Newsweek*. They decided that we had orchestrated the whole thing, that I had strung them along in my guidance, and that the inconvenience and expense they had suffered by holding their presses was the result of nothing more than our desire to make sure the announcement ceremony was a surprise and during prime time.

This particularly irritated me, since I had taken time during those hectic thirty minutes to give the *Newsweek* correspondents a quick call to let them know that the summit was ending as a success, thus enabling them to write a new and accurate lead for their summit story. Even after the papers began to print chronologies of the last hours at Camp David, which made it clear that the issue had been in doubt until the last moment, a few anonymous Newsweekers from New York continued to grouse to reporters about "media extravaganzas" and "playing to the networks." Their real problem was, of course, the almighty dollar.

However, in the jubilation of the moment, and in keeping with my earlier determination to view the vicissitudes of the job with greater equanimity, I let the matter pass. It was a time to be savored and to bask in the warm glow of success. Had I realized how short that time would be, I would have been even less inclined to mar it with recriminations.

FROM CAMP DAVID TO CAIRO

W hat we had after Camp David was a framework for a peace treaty and a great deal of goodwill, plus extremely high expectations. By November of 1978, the goodwill had largely dissipated, the framework itself appeared to be in danger, and the high expectations were beginning to create political problems as it became clear to the public that translating that framework into an actual treaty of peace would be a long and difficult task.

In that time period Prime Minister Begin had announced plans for new West Bank settlements, disputed our interpretation of some of what had been agreed to at Camp David, and talked of moving his office to East Jerusalem.

On the Arab side, the Saudis had, publicly at least, thrown in with the hardliners and Hussein was soon to follow suit.

Visits back and forth by Foreign Ministers failed to make any progress in the months that followed. We were becoming convinced that events were again working against us, and unless the agreement on a peace treaty could quickly be made final, all the progress at Camp David would evaporate.

Nor was this the only problem on the President's plate: the democratic midterm conference convened in December, furnishing a forum for the President's critics from within his own party. Vice-President Mondale warned them prophetically, and in vain, that unless they supported the President's austerity measures, inflation would sweep Democrats from office in 1980.

But labor leaders from George Meany on down rejected the

President's call for voluntary wage and price restraint. Three years later, many of the same leaders who had denounced the idea of a 7 percent *increase* in wages would meekly accept *cuts* in wages of several times that amount as tens of thousands of their members stood in the unemployment lines.

The Shah of Iran was tottering on the Peacock Throne. He would seek our advice, refuse to act, and fall—with profound consequences for the American economy and the political future of the Carter administration.

A new budget was prepared and proposed amid the crosscurrents of rising inflation and declining economic growth.

A brief spell of optimism in the negotiations over the future of Namibia quickly dissipated. (At this writing those negotiations are still in progress with little hope of success in the near future.)

Normalization of relations with China was announced at year's end, changing the strategic map of the world and provoking a prolonged and bitter struggle with the Republican right wing in Congress and the courts.

That diplomatic coup and the subsequent visit of Chinese leader Deng Xiaoping to Washington was the occasion for an amusing incident that had nothing to do with the Middle East and a lot to do with my attitudes toward the more pretentious pundits in American journalism, of which there are more than a few.

The social highlight of the Vice-Chairman's visit was a gala to be held at the Kennedy Center on the evening of January 29, 1979. All of Washington and a good portion of the rest of the country were scrambling for tickets.

I managed to secure a dozen or so for the press, which raised the problem of how to distribute them. It seemed to me that first call ought to go to those who covered the President and the White House regularly, who had watched and reported daily on the work that had made this all possible. Included in that list were also some of the State Department correspondents who had been following the developments closely.

That seemed to work fine until the day of the gala. On that morning, syndicated columnist Joe Kraft began calling members of the President's senior staff. He was distraught. He had not, he said, gotten an invitation to the gala. It was a terrible embarrassment to him. He was not about to call that Jody Powell in the press office because he had probably been the one who took his name off the invitation list anyway. Could anyone help him?

When the staffers called me, I explained what I had done. I had no more tickets, but said that I would not object if Anne Wexler, a member of the White House senior staff who also had some to distribute to the leaders of various interest groups, wanted to find one for Joe.

That she did and called Kraft to give him the good news. Would she be so kind as to have them sent to his office by messenger? Mr. Kraft had a very busy day. She did.

An hour or two later, Kraft called back. There must have been some mistake. These tickets were in the balcony. Everyone he knew of any importance was going to be sitting down front. It would be almost as embarrassing to be seen in the balcony seats as not to go at all. By this time Anne's patience was running a bit thin. She explained that it was getting a bit late and tickets were in great demand, but she would see what could be done.

With some effort, she was able to find two more tickets for Mr. Kraft and his wife and called back to report her success. Mr. Kraft had left the office, but could be reached at home.

When reached at home, Joe wanted to know if the tickets could be sent out by White House messenger.

By now it was late in the afternoon. The tickets were already at the Kennedy Center. A messenger might not have time to pick them up and get to the Krafts' house before they would need to leave. Could he pick them up at the "will call" office and drop off the two in the balcony?

That was such a hassle, but he guessed it would be all right.

Shortly after eight that evening, the President and Vice-Chairman Deng were about to enter the presidential box for the opening of the gala. Down below, about halfway back in the center of the orchestra section, were two vacant seats. Joe and Polly Kraft had failed to show. There were also two vacant seats in the balcony, the original Kraft tickets that had not been returned for someone else to use.

Even during the Deng visit the President was unable to put the Middle East completely aside. In the weeks that followed, the Bakhtiar government fell in Iran to be replaced by Khomeini's religious fanatics, the American embassy in Tehran was briefly overrun by an Iranian mob and quickly cleared, and the People's Republic of China went to war with the Socialist Republic of Vietnam. But always there was the Middle East and never did there seem to be any sign of real progress.

Deng and his Chinese delegation were hardly out of town before Prime Minister Begin and the Israelis were on their way. It was that singularly unproductive series of meetings with Prime Minister Begin and his advisers in late February and early March of 1979 that prompted the President to go to the Middle East in a last-ditch, personal effort to put together a peace treaty. He had virtually concluded, I think, before ever discussing it with the rest of us, that this was his only chance of salvaging what had begun at Camp David.

I first learned of what he was planning on the morning of March 3. It was a surprise to me and an unpleasant one. I agreed that there was a need for forceful action, but setting sail for Cairo and Jerusalem on short notice was not at all what I had in mind.

I did not want my concerns about press relations to become a dominant factor, but I thought they should be put on the table.

We would, I argued, have none of the advantages everyone agreed had been such a help at Camp David. We would be on their turf, not ours. The control of leaks would be virtually impossible, and the pressure for Sadat and Begin to posture would be even greater in their own capitals than in Washington.

To make matters worse, I said, there was no possible way to arrange the logistics of such a trip adequately in the time between that moment and when the President wanted to arrive.

Foreign trips under the best of circumstances greatly complicate press relations, particularly with a President like Carter, who insisted on maintaining a whirlwind schedule. The working days for reporters, and thus the press office staff, seem never to end.

If you are in Jerusalem, for example, the day begins on Jerusalem time, five hours earlier than in Washington. But it does not end until the final deadlines are past back in the States. If you work for a network, the evening news deadline is not five-thirty or six in the afternoon but ten-thirty or eleven that night. The Washington edition of the *New York Times* can take copy until eleven at night. And if you work for the *Los Angeles Times*, you could be pounding away at a story until two in the morning Jerusalem time.

That is on a normal trip. On this one, the schedule would certainly be even more frantic. There might or might not be time to set up all the communications facilities that allow the press to file easily and the press office to keep in touch with what the President and his people are doing. There was some question about whether we would even be able to get all the press in the same hotel.

All of this would add significantly to the frustration and fatigue that are always present. In such an atmosphere, innocent mistakes on both sides of the podium are more likely to occur. Furthermore, tired and irritable staffers' dealings with tired and irritable journalists can result in errors of fact or interpretation that are not altogether innocent, and therefore more damaging.

The President listened to my arguments. But I could tell he was not particularly moved by them, and perhaps he should not have been. His job was to salvage what might be the last chance for real peace in the Middle East. If I could not figure out some way to get the press to cover such an effort fairly, that was my problem.

If my concerns had made any impression at all, it was totally erased the next day when the President spoke to Sadat. The Egyptian President had also reached the end of his tether. He wanted to come to Washington and denounce Begin for wrecking the work at Camp David. When the President told him about his thoughts on a personal trip to Egypt and Israel, Sadat's mood changed instantly. He was now optimistic and assured the President that his mission would be a success.

The President was inclined to read more into that assurance than I was. He was sure it meant that Sadat would bend over backward to keep the visit from being a failure. I thought it more likely that he was just being polite. What else was he going to say—"Come ahead, Mr. President, but I must tell you there is a good chance that your trip will be a disastrous failure"?

As it turned out, the President had read his friend Anwar Sadat much better than I.

By the time the final decision was announced and our advance teams were dispatched, there were only five days before the

President's arrival in Cairo. I had also learned that the visit would include a trip to Alexandria, by train, no less. Under normal circumstances, five weeks would have been considered too short a time to prepare for such a trip.

But times were not normal, and everyone seemed to know it. The advance operation did a magnificent job. The first day or so was rough, but then things settled down. Even the press griped much less than I had expected about the foul-ups and inconveniences that continued to crop up.

I will not bore the reader with a blow-by-blow account of the negotiations; others more directly involved than I have written on that subject. Suffice it to say that by the time we left Cairo the President and his advisers were moderately optimistic. From our first day in Jerusalem that optimism began to wane. By the last night it had disappeared completely. Then, in a few hours it all turned around. And thereby hangs a tale.

Monday, March 12, was to be our last full day in Jerusalem. It was also the low point of the trip. The President had yet another nonproductive meeting with the Israeli Cabinet that morning, addressed the Knesset, and sent Secretary Vance back for one more session with the Cabinet.

Vance returned to the President's hotel, the King David, about 6:30 P.M. with a draft press release that had been handed to him that afternoon by the Israelis. It said that the talks had terminated after "further important progress . . . in the effort towards . . . an Egyptian-Israeli peace treaty. The President and the Prime Minister agreed on the ongoing need to continue the negotiations between Israel through the good offices of the United States."

Our worst suspicions were confirmed. The Israelis were prepared to leave it at that. They expected that Sadat and Carter would be content to go back to the prolonged and apparently stalemated negotiations. This was in direct conflict with our estimation of the situation. The President was convinced that Sadat's patience was running out. He had not come to the Middle East to make marginal and barely discernible progress, and he was not about to cooperate in trying to put the best possible face on what would quickly and correctly be viewed as a failed mission.

The mood during and after Vance's briefing of the President was somber, disappointment mixed with a touch of anger. The President decided that we should stay overnight, primarily because a departure that evening would seem ill mannered. He also called Prime Minister Begin and invited him to come by for a farewell breakfast the next morning. We would depart for Cairo, he said, around noon, and he would break the bad news to Sadat.

In the midst of the meeting, we learned that the Israelis were describing the results of our meetings in the most positive manner, further confirming our belief that they profoundly misunderstood the attitude of the United States and Egypt.

Shortly after the session, the President left for an already scheduled trip with Israeli archaeologist and peace proponent Yigael Yadin to see the Dead Sea Scrolls. I remained with Vance, Brzezinski, Jordan, and others who had been involved in the talks to discuss what I should say to the press that evening.

At eight I left the King David for the Jerusalem Hilton, where the press was staying and where the White House Press Office operation was located. I was greeted by Deputy Press Secretary Rex Granum, who said the press was all abuzz with the optimistic comments from Israeli spokesman Patir, who had briefed earlier that evening. The need to put things back into perspective was apparent.

Shortly before I walked out to begin the briefing, the phone in the press office rang. It was Hamilton, and he said I might want to know that Moshe Dayan had called Vance and asked if he could come over for an informal chat. Hamilton did not know what it meant, or whether Israeli Foreign Minister Dayan was acting on Begin's behalf, or even with his knowledge.

In fact, Dayan had been meeting with the Israeli Cabinet at the same time as the American delegation was meeting in the King David. They sensed serious trouble ahead and had come up with some last-minute ideas that they thought might be worth exploring. Dayan's mission was to try them out on Vance. If his response was positive, Vance was to try to ask the President to make another run at Begin the next morning.

After talking to Hamilton, I decided not to mention the Dayan-Vance meeting unless I was asked about it. I did not want the press flocking to the King David to try to catch him on the way out, particularly if he was there without Begin's knowledge. Even if I had known what was taking place at the meeting, which began about thirty minutes before I started my briefing, my pessimism would have been only slightly lessened. Dayan and Defense Minister Ezer Weizman were almost always more flexible than Begin. It was Begin who made the final decisions, and their ability to bring him along was a sometime thing at best.

My job at the briefing was delicate—to convey a sense of disappointment and impending failure without officially characterizing negotiations that had not yet been formally concluded. There was the breakfast meeting with Begin still to come, and Sadat deserved to hear an analysis directly from the President rather than indirectly through his press secretary.

Actually the task was not that difficult. After two years the White House correspondents had learned to read between the lines of my comments very well. They could be counted on to make sure the Israeli reporters who had not had as much practice got the message.

I opened the briefing by announcing that the President would be having breakfast with Prime Minister Begin in the morning and departing for Egypt shortly thereafter, where he would review his discussions in Israel with President Sadat. I refused to deny that I was "unhappy" with the outcome, although I took some of the edge off the response by wondering aloud what difference it made to anyone whether the press secretary was happy or not.

I also refused to comment on Prime Minister Begin's statement that "great progress" had been made. Throughout I made clear that I was not going to characterize the results of the visit, but suggested that the reporters draw their own conclusions.

I could sense that the effect of the earlier Israeli press briefing had been even stronger than I had expected. As the session began to draw to a close, I was not sure that I had yet gotten the message across, so I took advantage of a question on exactly what the President was going to say to Sadat:

"I hope you understand the position I am in. It is certainly not appropriate for me to say that . . . I see very little possibility that these issues are going to be resolved. There is always that possibility, of course, but I think you know enough about the process to know that that has not usually been the case in these discussions."

That did it. After a few more questions, the briefing ended at 10:17 P.M., Jerusalem time.

Thirty minutes later I was meeting with the American broadcast correspondents in a private room at the Jerusalem Hilton. This was a practice I had adopted on our first foreign trip. When overseas, I had to be even more careful than usual about what was said in the official briefings; there were always large numbers of foreign correspondents in attendance who were unfamiliar with my style and might misinterpret what I said, or even misunderstand because of language difficulties. I never spoke on "background" at such briefings because you could never be sure that the ground rule would be understood or honored.

At the closed sessions with the familiar White House crowd, we could all be more relaxed and I could speak more bluntly without fear of my comments being misused. That night, as was my usual practice, I met with the broadcast correspondents first because their deadlines were earlier and they needed less detail.

In this case, I told both groups essentially the same thing. After describing the issues that remained unresolved, and making it clear that even with the Dayan meeting and the Carter-Begin session in the morning I was not optimistic, I was asked how I would describe the situation if I had a story to write—exactly the sort of question that would never be asked in a formal briefing.

My answer would have been equally inappropriate in an official context. After kidding the correspondents about how much I hated to be in the position of telling them how to write their leads—a statement that they knew to be the exact opposite of the truth—I said that I suppose I would have to say that things did not look good at all, but it was the Middle East, so "you'd better cover your ass."

Later, when I met with the print reporters, I ended with the same advice in almost the very same words. Everyone heeded the first part of my advice, but unfortunately for me and for them, not all covered their rear ends.

The *New York Times* and the *Washington Post* did. Their stories contained phrases like "appears to be foundering" and "no plan . . . and unresolved issues still remaining . . . unless Carter can reverse [the situation] with a last-minute success." The *Washington Star*, being an afternoon paper, was able to have the later, and official, announcement for most of its editions. But the *Los Angeles Times* went a bit further. The President was described as "abandoning his hope of winning Israeli and Egyptian agreement to a treaty package." Fortunately, there was a brief mention of the "faint hope" that the meetings still to be held "could salvage matters."

Among the networks, ABC was the most cautious, reporting that the President's day had been "ambiguous." NBC was almost as wary, saying that the mission was close to an end with no final agreement reached. CBS was farthest out on the limb with hindquarters fully exposed, saying, "All indications are that Carter's Mideast gamble has failed." Later, Cronkite described the President's speech to the Knesset as sounding as though he "had just seen his diplomatic house of cards collapse."

Both wire services straddled the fence rather well in their stories for morning papers. Unfortunately, they had to write for the afternoon papers that same night from the same information. Frank Cormier of the Associated Press, one of the most experienced, hardworking, and decent of all the reporters covering the White House, decided to roll the dice. He knew his story would be appearing in papers that were hitting the streets in the United States just as the President was departing Cairo. By then, everyone would know for sure what the outcome was; he could not, would not have them reading an "on the one hand, on the other hand" story from the AP. He led his story for the P.M. papers with a flat statement that the President's mission had failed and went on to explain the reasons for this depressing turn of events.

Needless to say, when the President walked to the podium at the Cairo airport the next day to announce that an agreement had been reached, Mr. Cormier had mixed emotions. I did not realize quite how mixed until several hours later when I boarded the press plane for the return to Washington.

Because of the fast-paced and uncertain schedule of the trip, we had not been able to arrange for filing facilities at the airport. We had to drive into Cairo to the Nile Hilton and reactivate the press room we had abandoned three days earlier. Fortunately, our press advance people had had the foresight to keep the telephone and Telex lines in place.

My briefing there only added to the irritation of those who felt they had been misled and embarrassed. There was almost nothing in the way of usable information.

The problem was that I did not know exactly what had happened that morning to turn defeat into victory. The few who did know were all on Air Force One with the President discussing the next step, and there had been no time to debrief them on the short flight from Jerusalem to Cairo because they had been meeting to plan how to approach Sadat.

I was reluctant to discuss what little I did know because the agreement was much more tentative than it had been at Camp David. Nothing had been signed. The entire agreement still had to be approved by the Israeli parliament. I was determined that if there was nothing I could do to be helpful, I could at least make sure that I did not cause any problems.

Running constantly through my mind was the fear that I might touch on some sensitive area that would provoke denials and recriminations from one side or the other. If that happened, the President would land at Andrews only to discover that his hard-won agreement had come unraveled because of his press secretary's big mouth.

I need not have worried. Rereading the transcript of that briefing, even now I find it a model of double-talk and noninformation.

I was not happy with my briefing, but I was still exhilarated by the sudden breakthrough. As I boarded the plane for the return to Washington, I was looking forward to a cold drink, a good dinner, and a few hours of sleep. Seated in the row across from me was the gentlemanly Frank Cormier. He was not in a gentle mood.

He looked at me with an expression of unspeakable pain and disillusionment and said, "My press secretary has lied to me. I trusted him and he lied to me."

From there the conversation quickly went downhill. It lasted the better part of two hours, and touched upon such subjects as the punishments that await untrustworthy spokesmen in this world and the next, the general reputation and specific sexual idio-

syncrasies of the Powell and Cormier families for several genera-
tions back, and the just deserts of journalists who fail to cover
their asses after being specifically warned to do so and then try to
lay the blame on an honest, hardworking public servant.

The exchange was witnessed by a growing crowd of journalists and press office staffers whose reactions moved from interest,
to horror, and then to amusement as the libations dispensed by
the Pan Am crew began to dull our wits, if not our emotions.

Four years later, Cormier has mellowed on this subject, but
not a lot. It was, he says, my job to make myself understood.
Whatever my reasons, and he now admits that there may not have
been any intent to deceive, I had sent at least some reporters away
with a mistaken impression. That is an argument that is hard to
dispute.

Cormier also agrees, grudgingly, that it is part of a reporter's
job to make sure he understands. There, I suspect, is the best
place to let the matter rest.

When I got back to Andrews, I discovered that CBS's people
were very upset at having gone out on the limb as far as they had.
They expressed their pique on the evening news. Their coverage
was as negative as possible for a story about a peace treaty between Israel and Egypt.

Their lead described the President's statement at the airport
as "mildly optimistic" and "clearly designed to put pressure on
Israel."

Then there was a report that the treaty would cost the American taxpayers "$10 billion over the next few years, and be the
single most costly effort in U.S. history." The figure was as
wildly inflated as the rhetoric.

Finally, there was a report by Lesley Stahl enumerating a list
of charges from anonymous Israeli officials. The allegations were
false and ambiguous, and would hardly have been newsworthy
except they just happened to exonerate CBS for going out on the
limb the night before.

The United States, according to this report, had "distorted
facts" as part of a plan "orchestrated by Jerry Rafshoon to make it
look as though the President had performed a miracle." We had, it
was claimed, lied about the morning meeting with Begin, saying

that it was a courtesy call and that the talks were "virtually over" when we "knew full well that meeting was crucial."

Not only were the allegations untrue, but most of them were obviously unknowable to any Israeli official inasmuch as they dealt with the attitudes and state of mind of American officials. How on earth could an Israeli official know what role Jerry Rafshoon, the President's friend and media analyst, had played in my briefing? As a matter of fact, he had played none.

The CBS coverage that evening is noteworthy because it combined several of the most unattractive characteristics of American journalism at its worst.

First, there was the familiar touch of arrogance, the absolute refusal to admit that a mistake has been made. If something is wrong, it must, by definition, be someone else's fault.

Then there was the less common but more serious practice of publicizing unsupported allegations that are almost impossible to prove or to refute—often based on anonymous sources. Stahl closed her piece by admitting that she did not know whether there was any truth to the charges. It amounted to little more than saying, "CBS would like you to know that certain Israeli officials say that the American government is being run by liars and schemers of the first order. We have no way of determining whether that is true, but wanted you to know about it anyway."

Although this type of story is by no means an everyday occurrence, it is more common than most journalists like to admit. Six months later CBS did it again, with accusations about Hamilton Jordan and drug use, with more serious consequences.

Finally, this was a classic example of the use of the tremendous power and privileges accorded the news media for essentially self-serving purposes, a practice that produces screams of self-righteous indignation from journalists when indulged in by other institutions. A significant portion of the CBS Mideast reporting on that Tuesday evening was devoted to covering its rear end because it had failed to do so on the preceding evening.

To be fair to other news outlets, it should be noted that both the *Washington Post* and the *Washington Star* did stories the next day that reconstructed the events of that last night in Jerusalem and concluded that there had been no intent to deceive.

Also in the interest of fairness, it should be pointed out that I could have done a better job that evening. However, I would not change anything I said during the official briefing or the backgrounders that followed. My mistake was in what I did afterward—which was nothing.

After my session with Cormier on the press plane, I was told by Rex Granum that Ozzie Johnston of the *Los Angeles Times* was also upset. I walked back to talk to him about his grievances. He was clearly not happy, but neither was he in the mood to argue. "Why," he said, "didn't you check with someone and find out whether the Vance-Dayan meeting had raised any new possibilities?" A good question for which there is no good answer.

By the time the background briefings were finished, any new information would have been useless to the networks for evening news, and to most of the morning papers, whose deadlines were already past. Nor was there anything definite to report. But had I talked with one of the officials involved at that very moment in drafting new proposals for the meeting with Prime Minister Begin the next morning, I would have discovered that the mood had changed, not significantly, but measurably; and the nuances of mood were exactly what I was dealing with that night. With that information, I could have helped Johnston, whose West Coast paper has later deadlines, Cormier on his P.M. story, and even the networks for their morning shows. They could have at least reported that U.S. officials had been up all night working on last-ditch proposals to break the impasse.

I did not make the call primarily because I did not think anyone would still be awake at the King David. I had reconciled myself to the idea that the trip would end in failure. But there was also another reason. Sam Donaldson was being given a surprise birthday party that night at the press hotel. Any party with Sam is a memorable occasion, and on that night I felt badly in need of distraction. So I went partying instead of finishing my job.

As is usually the case, the person who suffered most from my mistakes and the shortcomings of the press was the President. Although CBS was the most negative, the coverage generally in the days that followed was not good. The focus was on the cost in increased aid and on all the things that could go wrong and on the problems yet to be solved.

On March 15 the *Washington Post* carried stories headlined

THE PRICE OF PEACE $5 BILLION IN AID and TREATY SEEN STRAINING U.S. RELATIONSHIP WITH OTHER ARAB COUNTRIES.

The same day the *New York Times* headlined the price of peace as being only $4 billion. Its lead editorial, which was headed THE THEATER OF PEACE, fretted about the spectacle of "foreign ministers taking the role of messengers and heads of government performing as scribes." The "dramatics" (never let it be said that the *Times* fails to sustain its metaphors) had given rise to "terrible distortions." "The price of Sinai oil or the date for exchange of Ambassadors" had been allowed to loom larger than more important matters. Indeed, the *Times* concluded, "the Carter Administration gave far from a flawless performance in this drama," but deserved a pat on the head anyway.

The reporting and analysis on costs, pitfalls, and difficulties were not particularly inaccurate, but were unbalanced by any attention to the benefits of what had happened. We were never able to get anyone to report how much aid was already going to Israel, which would have put the increase in better perspective, or to make a comparison between the increased aid and the cost of another war.

In part the negativism was a reaction to the excessive euphoria that had followed Camp David, only to be quickly tarnished by months of bickering and stalemate. But it was also a consequence of the feeling, or at least the suspicion, among many journalists that they had somehow been manipulated on that last night in Jerusalem—a feeling that I might have prevented.

In this case the results could also be precisely measured, in at least one area. Shortly after the signing of the peace treaty, Pat Caddell's polls showed that the President had gotten no benefit in the minds of the public from his accomplishment. His approval ratings had hardly moved at all. The networks, and to a lesser extent the print press, had succeeded in convincing the American public that one of the most dramatic and important diplomatic triumphs in recent American history was seriously flawed—too fragile, too expensive, with much less to it than met the eye.

If it is indeed the good things we do but receive no credit for that are of greatest benefit to our immortal souls, the fourth estate was responsible in four short years for the laying up of a wealth of benefits for the soul of James Earl Carter. Unfortunately, sometimes his press secretary helped out, too.

A GRAVE
MISTAKE_____

One of the dangers in writing a book about events in which one played a role is that there inevitably comes the point where a decision must be made about how to deal with your own behavior. The decision is particularly difficult if the action in question may be seen by some as ill advised, or even downright stupid.

Will you be as brutal in describing and assessing the consequences of your own actions as you have been of others'? Or will you yield to the temptation to leave out the most embarrassing details?

We have now come to such a point in this revisitation of the relationship between the Carter White House and the press. I would be less than honest if I failed to admit that the temptation is great to follow the traditional pattern established by Washington books, and those written by White House aides in particular. In such an approach, the primary goal is to establish the wisdom and good intentions of the author, usually at the expense of his or her colleagues. If it can be at the expense of the President, so much the better.

At its most refined, the model goes something like this:

> The President was clearly troubled when he walked into the Cabinet room that morning. The difficult choices before him had apparently disturbed his sleep. [This line can be safely used with all Presidents except the present one.]
> After looking slowly around the Cabinet table, he turned

to me—as he often did in such situations. "What shall we do?" he asked.

"Mr. President," I said calmly, "given the responsibilities of the office you hold and your sworn duty to protect and defend the Constitution of this country, you have only one option.

"Do not be tempted," I continued, my voice rising and deepening slightly [in case someone wants to make a movie of this, the "rising and deepening" part is important]. "Do not be tempted to follow the path of political expediency. Do not place your personal ambitions above the good of this nation, which we all love so dearly. Should you do such a thing, some of us would have no choice but to resign our positions and submit our dissent to the court of public opinion."

A hush fell over the room as I concluded my comments. No one, least of all I, knew how this vain and sometimes unpredictable man would react to my heartfelt but audacious challenge. The leader of the free world lowered his head for a moment. Then, looking me square in the eye, he said (as he often did in such situations), "Thanks, I needed that. You are right, of course."

And so it was that the Republic was saved, hungry children fed, and the world spared the horrors of nuclear war.

I personally have no doubt that the Republic has indeed been saved as frequently as, and in the precise manner, described in the hundreds of books by former White House aides, advisers, and domestic staff. I only wish that my behavior in the matter now before us had lived up to the high standards of those distinguished and patriotic men and women. Sadly, it did not.

The tragic incident to which I refer, as you may have already guessed, is the "killer rabbit" story.

It began late one afternoon in the spring of 1979. The President was sitting with a few of us on the Truman Balcony. He had recently returned from a visit to Plains, and we were talking about homefolks and how the quail were nesting and similar matters of international import.

Suddenly, for no apparent reason—he was drinking lemonade as I remember—the President volunteered the information that while fishing in a pond on his farm he had sighted a large animal swimming toward him. Upon closer inspection, the animal turned out to be a rabbit. Not one of your cutesy, Easter Bunny–type rabbits, but one of those big splay-footed things that we called swamp rabbits when I was growing up.

The animal was clearly in distress, or perhaps berserk. The President confessed to having had limited experience with enraged rabbits. He was unable to reach a definite conclusion about its state of mind. What was obvious, however, was that this large, wet animal, making strange hissing noises and gnashing its teeth, was intent upon climbing into the presidential boat. (As insightful columnists and congressional leaders later pointed out, none of this would have happened to the President if he had been sipping cocktails with them on the presidential yacht *Sequoia* like Presidents are supposed to do, instead of fishing in some godforsaken south Georgia swamp. But Carter had sold the *Sequoia,* and so being attacked by a rabbit was the least he deserved.)

Had I been doing my job, I would have stopped the President at that moment, pointed out the dangers to him and his administration if such a story ever got out, and sworn him and all within reach of his voice to secrecy.

Sadly, I did nothing of the kind. What is worse, and it still makes my flesh crawl to think I could have been so foolish, I thought it was funny. Can you imagine such a thing? Faced with a mortal threat to the Carter presidency, I laughed. Nor, as painful as it is to admit, was that the full extent of my culpability in this matter. The worst is yet to come.

Several months later I was chatting with Brooks Jackson, one of the White House correspondents for the Associated Press, over a cup of tea, as I remember. For reasons that I still do not fully understand, I told him about the President and the rabbit. I was the one who leaked the killer rabbit story.

Although an experienced reporter, Brooks also failed to appreciate the significance of what he had heard. He did not rush out to file an "urgent" story. In fact, he continued the conversation for some period of time and several more cups of tea. Not until the next day did he get around to sending this gripping account out over the wires to a waiting public. And even then it was a pleasant, lighthearted piece. Although he may not admit it now, I had the definite impression at the time that Brooks thought it was nothing more than a mildly amusing incident, too.

We were soon corrected. The *Washington Post*, exercising the news judgment that we in the White House had come to appreciate so keenly, headed the piece PRESIDENT ATTACKED BY RABBIT and ran it on the front page. The more cautious *New York Times* boxed it on page A-12. That night, all three networks found time to report the amazing incident. But that was just the beginning.

The nation's capital was shocked, incredulous. At Georgetown dinner parties the conversation focused on little else, and it was hushed, concerned, almost fearful. Bright young congressional aides could be seen scurrying through the halls of the Capitol, their earnest little brows deeply furrowed. Columnists and editorial writers waxed indignant:

What was to be done about a President with whom a rabbit would try to get into a boat? What did this startling, not to say worrisome, incident say about his fitness for office? What would the Russians think, not to mention the Cubans, the Ethiopians, and SWAPO?

A few months later, columnist George Will reportedly told friends that the President's timid response to the attack—he had shooed the rabbit away by splashing water at it with his paddle, rather than having the brute shot by the Secret Service—had led directly to the assault on our embassy in Tehran.

Columnist Robert Novak claimed to have seen communications intercepts that proved the invasion of Afghanistan was also a direct result of the incident.

The Reverend Jerry Falwell is said to have pointed out to associates that swamp rabbits were never mentioned in Revelation except in connection with Satan, and suggested that any true, heterosexual, right-thinking Christian would have seized upon this God-given opportunity to ruthlessly destroy this symbol of the Beast.

At the other end of the spectrum, Mary McGrory let it be known that she considered the brandishing of the paddle to be a clear example of excessive force. Why, she wondered, had the President not tried to engage the rabbit in constructive dialogue? Was not the boat big enough for both of them to share? Was this the sort of behavior that we should accept from the man whose finger was on the nuclear trigger? And what about Vietnam?

Covering both ends of the spectrum, Joseph Kraft is said to have reported gravely that three Prime Ministers, a King, a deposed dictator, and the entire board of directors of "big America"—with whom he was on the most intimate terms—had called to discuss the implications of this fiasco.

Hugh Sidey, distracted by the rejection of his proposed *Hugh Sidey–Betty Beale Report* by PBS, mailed his RABBITS HAVE NO CLASS column to the White House and published his letter imploring the President to meet with a group of *Time* magazine's principal advertisers. Sidey noted that this distinguished group had just returned from a round-the-world tour, during which they had dined with all the same people who had called Joe Kraft.

The *New Republic* declared forthrightly that Carter's attempt to beat the rabbit to death with a boat paddle was an indication of what he would do to Israel if he was elected to a second term.

In similar fashion, the *Boston Globe* suggested that this aquatic incident would quickly drive memories of Chappaquiddick from the minds of American voters, thus clearing the way for their Teddy to reclaim the family estate on Pennsylvania Avenue.

It was a nightmare. The story ran for more than a week. The President was repeatedly asked to explain his behavior at town hall meetings, press conferences, and meetings with editors.

There was talk of a suit under the Freedom of Information Act to force release of the picture showing the President, paddle, and rabbit in close proximity.

Shortly after the Reagan administration took office, they stumbled upon a copy of the picture—apparently while searching for a foreign policy—and reopened the old wounds by releasing it to the press. I have heard, but cannot confirm, that a copy of candidate Reagan's briefing materials, which was tossed over the White House fence by an anonymous courier wearing a stocking over his head, revealed that an allusion to the rabbit incident had been considered for Mr. Reagan's closing statement in the debate.

Almost four years later, I sat down for a chat with the political editor of a major regional newspaper and the first question he asked was about the killer rabbit story. He said he considered it to be the beginning of the end for the Carter administration.

Looking back on it now, I still have trouble understanding exactly what happened. Not that I have any doubt that my judgment throughout was woefully flawed or any wish to escape blame for the consequences. Indeed, this confession (I have never before been able to tell the whole sad story) has been a cleansing and uplifting experience. I feel now, as I write this, that a great burden of guilt and self-recrimination has been lifted.

Still, there is the desire to fit it into some larger context, to place it within the ebb and flow of the American political process. The best I have been able to do—and I know it is inadequate, though some will say impertinent—is to conclude that by August, 1979, if the President had been set upon by a pack of wild dogs, a good portion of the press would have sided with the dogs and declared that he had provoked the attack.

PYRAMIDS
OF THE NILE _____

A principal subject of this book is the story of the charges that Hamilton Jordan used cocaine at a New York night-club. It is impossible, however, to deal thoroughly with the way the press and the White House handled the cocaine story without describing the context in which it appeared. What happened to Hamilton when he was charged with using cocaine had a great deal to do with what had already happened to him. Past injustices contributed to those that occurred in the cocaine story. And to be fair, mistakes in the White House, for which Hamilton and I must bear the responsibility, also played a role.

Reporters from print and broadcast say that Hamilton Jordan's reputation was an important factor in their treatment of the cocaine charges against him. Reporters and editors who were involved in the cocaine story say that what they had heard and read about Hamilton for two and one half years prior to the cocaine charges caused them to be skeptical, if not downright disbelieving, of his claims of innocence. Most admit that they thought he was probably guilty.

By the summer of 1979, Hamilton had come to be viewed by the large portion of Washington that did not know him personally as a politically astute ne'er-do-well. Looking back on that time, reporters remember two events as being primarily responsible for creating that image in their minds: an allegation that he had made an indecent remark and gesture toward the wife of the Egyptian ambassador, and a report that he had spat a drink on a young woman in a Washington bar. Some of them also recall charges that he and I had made anti-Semitic statements during a fight in the Congress about the sale of advanced fighter aircraft to Saudi Arabia and Egypt.

The evolution of the three stories says a great deal about how reputations are made and unmade by sloppy and sometimes malicious journalism.

The story involving the Egyptian ambassador's wife appeared in the *Washington Post* on December 18, 1977, in the "Style" section. It was part of an article about the strained relations between the Carter administration and "Washington Society." It attracted significant national attention.

In Washington, a town that revels in such nasty personal tidbits, the impact was even greater. As one reporter who worked on the cocaine story put it, "The Egyptian story gave Hamilton Jordan the reputation of being someone who made an ass out of himself in public and didn't worry too much about the impact of his behavior on the President or the administration."

For almost the entire first year of the administration, there had been rumblings around town that the "Carter crowd" was antisocial. Our failure to appear regularly at Washington social events was variously interpreted as being the result of an anti-Washington mindset, or not having anything suitable to wear.

Syndicated columnist Rowland Evans called a young member of the White House staff to invite him to dinner. After determining that he was married, the columnist asked if his wife was "presentable." The staffer, somewhat taken aback, finally managed to reply civilly that he thought she probably was. The columnist then graciously included the wife in the invitation.

In fact, most of us were anything but antisocial. Our failure to participate more vigorously on the dinner circuit was the result of a variety of factors, mostly benign.

The most important and universal of these was that we were caught up in our jobs to the point of being overwhelmed. There was so much to learn and so much to do that there never seemed to be much time for socializing.

There was also an element of suspicion involved, but of a different sort than was generally understood. We did not know the players in Washington. We were reluctant to get too close to individuals who might be looking for an improper entrée to the

President. (I had in the back of my mind a warning from my early days in the Georgia governor's office. An old hand had remarked, "You are going to be welcomed by a lot of people with their hands outstretched, and more than a few of them are literally going to have their hands out—for more than a handshake.") And, being younger than most of our predecessors, we were also more likely to have young children at home. Many of us had neglected our families during two long years of campaigning. Now, when we had any free time at all, we wanted to stay home.

Lastly, the typical Washington social event was not exactly our idea of great fun. We discovered later that most everyone else in town felt the same way. (We had failed to understand from the outset that these things were not supposed to be fun.)

Thus we gravitated toward more informal gatherings, small enough so that everyone could sit down and talk with everyone else. Not only did we feel more comfortable, it was the only kind of entertaining that fit our budgets. My wife once remarked that if we had to host a seated dinner for five tables of ten, she would have to put three of the tables upstairs in the bedrooms.

It must also be said that we failed to appreciate until too late the repercussions of our failure to socialize in the traditional Washington manner. We missed an opportunity to get to know Washington better and to separate the sheep from the goats. We failed to establish personal relationships with individuals who could have been helpful to us professionally, who would have been there to defend us against the rumors and half-truths that constantly circulate in the nation's capital. Part of Washington felt that we were being arrogant and interpreted each regret as a snub. Others were confirmed in their belief that the entire administration, or at least the White House, had been taken over by the Visigoths.

Sally Quinn's *Post* story brought the strained relations between Washington socialites and the Carter White House to the fore. It was primarily a compilation of quotes from anonymous Washingtonians bemoaning the absence of Carterites on the social circuit. Although spiced with the touches of cattiness that had become Ms. Quinn's trademark, it was harmless and even amusing in places until the last 3 of its 105 paragraphs.

There it was reported that Hamilton Jordan, while attending

a dinner party given by Barbara Walters, had turned to the wife of the Egyptian ambassador, "gazed at [her] ample front, pulled at her elasticized bodice and was prompted to say, loudly enough for several others to hear, 'I've always wanted to see the pyramids.'"

The wire services jumped on the story immediately and began spreading it around the country, along with our denial that any such thing had taken place.

I considered making an effort to contact those who had been seated at the table with Hamilton and Mrs. Ghorbal to obtain support for our denial, but decided it was best to let the story die, if it would. That decision was a mistake.

Although other news organizations did contact several, including Mrs. Ghorbal, and none remembered seeing or hearing any such thing, the story did not die. It became an indelible part of Hamilton Jordan's image and made him vulnerable to more serious allegations later. Many, including the reporters who worked on the cocaine story, did not remember reading the follow-up stories containing the exculpatory statements. Those who did recall the denials considered the "don't remember" comments to be polite evasions, which they sometimes are but were not in this instance.

Shelby Coffey, the editor of the "Style" section at the time the story appeared, says that he took note of the item before it was published but was assured by Ms. Quinn that it was accurate. He does not remember if he asked for the names of her sources. And he feels sure that he did not attempt to talk to them himself.

Coffey did not think it strange that the story contained no denial, or even a comment on the incident, from anyone at the White House. He says that Ms. Quinn told him that no one at the White House was willing to talk to her, which was true. She apparently did not tell him that our refusal to talk was in reference to the Washington socializing story as a whole. We never had a chance to comment on the allegation about Hamilton because we only became aware of it when we read it in the paper.

Coffey says if he had it to do over again, he would have checked the story more thoroughly, but that it did not seem that important at the time. That may well be true. But many at the *Post* have long believed that Sally Quinn's stories were never subjected to the same level of editorial supervision as those produced by other writers. Her relationship and subsequent marriage to *Post* Executive Editor Benjamin Bradlee made her copy sacrosanct, in their view.

How much truth there is in that is difficult to determine. Undoubtedly there is a certain amount of professional jealousy involved. Sally's stories did seem to be allowed to run much longer than those of other "Style" section writers. She had also become somewhat of a star and a social figure in her own right, but that prominence was only partially derivative from Bradlee.

Our decision not to talk to Sally Quinn was a mistake. It was provoked by a story on the President's secretary, Susan Clough, that had appeared a few weeks earlier. The story strongly implied that there was an intimate relationship between the President and Ms. Clough. The entire White House was outraged, but there was nothing that could be done. There was no explicit allegation to deny, and any comment on the carefully worded innuendos would have only made matters worse.

But I was more outraged than most. About three fourths of the way through the same story, Sally also "reported" that Susan Clough had gotten her job as the President's secretary by sleeping with me.

There was no substantiation and no attribution. There was not even an anonymous source. Nor had I even been given an opportunity to deny it. If I had, I would have explained that Susan had indeed worked for me in the governor's office in Atlanta, but that had been the extent of the relationship. In fact, Susan and I had not worked well together. For that reason I had not asked her to work in the campaign press operation. When the President-elect asked my opinion on hiring her as his personal secretary, I said that I had not been able to establish a satisfactory working relationship. I had also said, however, that the fault might have been mine, and he might have a different experience. Largely because Susan had often filled in for his secretary in the governor's office, the President decided that they could get along.

Because of the stir caused by the implications about the President, no one paid much attention to my problem. No one in the press ever asked about it. I was thankful for that, but no less angry and bitter against the *Post* and Sally Quinn. My wife was also less than thrilled, to say the least.

A few days later, when I heard that Sally was doing a story about the social life at the White House, I suggested that we have nothing to do with her. It was partially because of the insult to the President, but I cannot deny that the gratuitous insult to my family, not to mention Ms. Clough, played a role in my attitude.

Had I not allowed personal feeling to interfere with my professional judgment, I suspect that Sally's story would never have contained the three paragraphs about Hamilton. They were thrown in at the end and were much more vicious in tone and effect than anything else in the piece.

Even more to the point, Sally sent word while her story was in preparation that she had something damaging to Hamilton that would be included in the story if we continued to refuse to talk to her, although she did not say what.

I also suspect that if the editors at the *Post* had been faced with a strong and categorical denial before the story ran, they would have killed the Jordan reference. At the very least, they would probably have done a much more thorough job of checking it out.

Another story cited by some reporters as shaping their attitudes toward Hamilton, and to some extent toward me, occurred the summer before the cocaine allegations, in 1978.

We were in the midst of a tough and sometimes bitter fight to obtain congressional approval for the sale of F-15 fighter aircraft to Saudi Arabia and Egypt. It was the first time an American president had sought to sell such advanced weapons to an Arab nation, and the sale was vigorously opposed by the government of Israel and by many American supporters of Israel. The matter was delicate, because thoughtful people on both sides of the issue realized the danger that ugly sentiments could be aroused. The administration went out of its way to avoid statements that could stir the anti-Semitism that unfortunately still exists in our society. Most of the leaders of the opposition tried with equal sincerity to prevent the characterization of those who supported the sale as anti-Semitic or anti-Israel. Those efforts had been largely successful until the day of the vote.

Hamilton and I were listening to live coverage of the Senate debate over National Public Radio when we heard Cokie Roberts, an NPR congressional correspondent, state that there was great resentment among some senators over "anti-Semitic remarks made by Hamilton Jordan and Jody Powell."

We could not believe our ears. This was exactly the sort of thing we feared and had worked hard to prevent. We believed, rightly or not, that as southerners we were particularly vulnerable to this sort of accusation. Members of the White House senior staff had been warned, and ordered to warn their subordinates, about any statement or action that might be misinterpreted. We had even been careful in private not to participate in the rough humor and wisecracks about the opposition that is normally a part of a political fight.

I immediately placed a call to Cokie Roberts. When she could not be reached, I called Frank Mankiewicz, the president of National Public Radio. I was less than my usual combative self when I talked to Mankiewicz. He was a presidential appointee, and though he was not subject to removal without cause, I did not want my complaint to be misinterpreted. He promised to check into the matter and get back to me.

A few minutes later, Cokie returned my call. There was no way that she could feel that her job was threatened by a call from the White House, so I felt no restraint in letting her know exactly how upset I was. I angrily denied her story and asked what substantiation she had. She replied that she could not discuss her sources with me. I said I was not asking for names, but I thought I had a right to know where and when Hamilton and I were alleged to have made these remarks. How could we convincingly prove our innocence if there were no specifics to the allegations? She refused to say anything more than that she felt she had the information on good authority.

In the meantime, Hamilton had placed calls to important Jewish friends of the administration, including several who were fighting us on the military sales issue. He also contacted Frank Moore, the head of the White House Congressional Liaison Office, so that he and his people would not be blind-sided by the charges on the Hill.

The next day, the problem got worse. A story in the *New York Times*, written by Cokie's husband, Steve Roberts, repeated the allegations. Although more people probably heard the NPR report than read the *Times* story, the latter was more serious. It gave currency and legitimacy to the charges. They became part of the semi-official record. Historians and reporters rehashing the vote years later would turn to the *New York Times* clips, now available to researchers on computer, and learn that senior staff members for the first President from the Deep South in more than a hundred years had attempted to appeal to bigotry in a fight over arms sales to the Middle East.

The immediate impact was also greater. Not everyone who was politically influential in Washington had heard the NPR story, but they all read the *New York Times*.

A few other news organizations had called to check on Cokie's allegations, and so far as I could determine, none had repeated them following our denial. Mr. Roberts had not bothered to check.

When I called Steve, he adopted the same position as his wife: he had to protect his sources and would not go beyond what had appeared in the paper.

My second call to Mankiewicz was even more disappointing and irritating. He said he had checked with his reporter and she had assured him that her story was accurate. I asked if he had spoken personally with her source or sources. He had not. I asked if he had even asked for the names of those sources. He had not. His attitude was "You just have to trust your reporters. If she's satisfied, so am I."

After pleading with him again to check for himself before he made up his mind to let the story stand and being refused, I told him that his position was the most ridiculous bunch of crap I had ever heard, particularly from someone who had been on the other side of the fence and ought to know better.

I had never run into a news executive who refused to check into the sourcing of a story. (My attitude toward Mankiewicz would never be the same after that incident.) I ended the conversation with the mental resolve to have nothing further to do with him unless it was absolutely necessary. As it turned out, I spoke with Frank only once more during the remaining two and one half years of the administration.

My next call to Cokie was a little more productive. She relented somewhat in her refusal to discuss the story and told me that the remarks had been made at a cocktail party within the past week or ten days. I told her that I had not been to a cocktail party in the past two weeks, and after buzzing Hamilton reported that he had not either. I asked her to go back to her source and find out where and on what nights this alleged party had taken place. Thoroughly angry by this point, I also asked that she tell her source that I said he was a bald-faced liar and was prepared to prove it if he would stand up and make his charges on the record so he could be cross-examined.

A few days later, Connie Lawn, a free-lance reporter who was covering the arms sale fight for the Israeli national radio, came in to see me. She was visibly upset and extremely apologetic. She had run essentially the same story. Her source was the same as Cokie's. When she went back to him, he was unable to give any specific persons, places, or dates for the remarks. She concluded that she had been misled.

Connie asked that I not reveal the substance of her conversation with me, but I felt free to use it to challenge the story without mentioning her name. I called Cokie, Steve, and Mankiewicz and told them that I had heard from another reporter who had run the same story, but was convinced that there was no substance to it. All three refused to discuss the matter further, and neither NPR nor the *New York Times* ever made any further effort to set the record straight except to report that Hamilton and I had denied making any anti-Semitic remarks.

Much later I was informed, by one in a position to know, that the source for both Cokie and Connie was Morris Amitay, then executive director of the American Israeli Public Affairs Committee, the principal group lobbying against the arms sale. However, he denies that he ever said any such thing to anyone.

TRASH
IN JOURNALISM_____

Despite the small-town background of many of us in the Carter administration, we were not prepared for the Washington brand of talebearing when we came to town. Nor were we prepared for the relationship between what some people call news and others call gossip.

In Washington, as in small towns, the purveyors of gossip are well known to the community. They have no trouble finding an eager audience. In small towns, however, that audience is small enough to be manageable. It is limited by the number of phones on a party line, chairs at the beauty parlor, and guests at a bridge party. The victim has at least a fifty-fifty chance to catch up with the rumor and correct the record. False witness is a common sin, but its effects are usually short-lived.

In Washington, the audience is limited only by the spread of the English language. The party line has been replaced by network television; the beauty parlor and the bridge party have given way to the newsrooms of national and international publications.

In a small town some of the dirt inevitably rubs off on those who traffic in it. The status and reputation of the chief gossip is always a bit lower than it otherwise would have been. The practice of this ancient avocation always constitutes a step down for the practitioner. Gossip mongering in a small town is considered a tolerable weakness in character, ranking somewhere between alcoholism and promiscuity in the hierarchy of transgressions. Gossips are invited to social occasions or into one's home in spite of their shortcoming.

In Washington they are on the invitation list because of it. Gossip is an avenue to high status and even higher income. The most accomplished practitioners are better paid than a United States senator or the speaker of the House.

The other principal difference is that small-town gossips are, on the whole, more concerned with the truth.

My own family got its first taste of how the gossip game is played in Washington in the spring of 1977, when a neighbor called to report that she had witnessed a strange event. At dawn on a Thursday morning, a small car pulled to the curb beside our house and a young man jumped out, placed two vinyl bags of garbage in the backseat, and sped off.

At first we were amused. I was not worried that some sensitive document had been discarded by mistake. I had long ago developed the practice of almost never bringing work home. For me it was better to stay at the office as long as necessary to finish whatever needed to be done, and leave the papers and the worries behind when I headed home.

The only other person we had ever heard of who had had his garbage stolen was Henry Kissinger. But he was the architect of American foreign policy. Issues of war and peace were involved. Who ever heard of sorting through the domestic leavings of a White House flack?

But a few days later the phone calls began to come in. My wife received a call from Helen Cleaveland, a friend from Atlanta who had recently been transferred to Washington. Helen said she had just had an unusual conversation with one Jay Gourley of the *National Enquirer*, who wanted to know about the affair she was having with me. A piece of paper with the name Helen, the name of her company, and a phone number had been in the garbage that night. It had been written by my wife. At the time I did not even know that the lady the *Enquirer* was pairing me with was in town.

Two days later we learned that the pastor of a church we had visited had also been called by Mr. Gourley. This time he wanted to know about the "counseling sessions" the minister had been having with our daughter Emily.

What was the purpose of this counseling? What problems did

Mr. Powell's daughter have, and what newsworthy crisis might she be facing? Were there drugs involved?

A letter from the pastor inviting us back to church had been in the stolen garbage. It was addressed to Emily because she had signed the visitor's card, and it contained a short handwritten note saying he had enjoyed the chance to talk with her. The talk had taken place at the door of the church at the end of the morning service.

In our case, Mr. Gourley's effort was for naught. His calls to creditors—Nan had paid the bills the night before I put the garbage on the curb—and to friends turned up no juicy tidbits. So far as I know, our trash bags produced no story for the *National Enquirer*.

In some ways that first experience was misleading. In the coming years we found that sifting through garbage in search of a story is not confined to employees of the *National Enquirer*, and some news organizations that turn up their noses at the *Enquirer* are less careful about checking the accuracy of the trash that comes in over the telephone than Mr. Gourley was with what he picked up from the street.

* * * * *

And whosoever shall offend one of these little ones . . . , it is better for him that a millstone were hanged about his neck, and he were cast into the sea.

Nothing during the entire four years of the Carter administration left me more bitter, nor with a more abiding revulsion for those responsible, than the way Amy Carter was treated by some in the press. I should hasten to add that in this case I am referring to a very small minority of journalists. Most of those who covered the White House, whatever their feelings about the administration, were too mature to take out their differences on a child; and they shared, to some extent, my contempt for the few who did.

If I have a complaint against that majority, it is that they kept their condemnation to themselves. Never was I able to get any one of them to say in print or on the air what they were quite willing to say privately.

That feeling of cold, impotent fury that is as fresh and real as

I write this today as it was six years ago was shared by most of my colleagues in the White House, particularly those of us who had watched Amy grow from a little girl to an adolescent now approaching young womanhood. Our feelings were further inflamed, to the extent that was possible, because many of us had children of our own. Frank Moore, Zbigniew Brzezinski, Jim McIntyre, Jack Watson, and I—to mention just a few—all had daughters of about the same age as Amy.

If it is natural, at least in the old-fashioned sense, for fathers to feel especially protective of daughters, it is as inevitable to feel particularly sympathetic with the same emotions in other fathers. In this case, the other father was our boss and the President of the United States; but that had little to do with the way we or he felt at the time.

I had always assumed that those who treated Amy so cruelly must have no children of their own. Surely no one who had ever experienced that intense desire to protect a child from harm could so casually and callously inflict it. In researching this book, I found that I was wrong. Some of these journalists have children of their own. Either they have long since lost whatever nurturing instinct they once had, or perhaps all they learned from the experience was how deeply you can wound a parent by hurting the child.

I should make clear that my complaint here is not against the routine buffeting that children of any person in public life receive. It cannot be pleasant for any child to see a parent pilloried in the press. And other children, as the old saying goes, can be extraordinarily mean in such situations. That, however, is an inescapable correlate of public life, a burden that one knowingly imposes on spouse and children when the decision to pursue such a career is made.

(I do think, however, that it would be worthwhile for journalists to bear in mind that when they falsely accuse someone of wrongdoing, the damage that is done is not confined to the one accused. The pain and embarrassment and scars are borne by the entire family, including the children.)

My outrage here is directed toward those so-called journalists who attack the parent through the child, who are so bent upon doing harm to an adult—or on selling a story or a column—that they are completely willing to attack children if that is what it takes to get the job done. No more repugnant creatures exist on the face of the earth.

For those who may think my earlier comments about old-fashioned fathers a bit sexist, I will now compound the offense by admitting that it was always particularly hard for me to accept the fact that the writer who was by far the most vicious to Amy was a woman.

In March of 1978, Diana McClellan was writing a gossip column called "The Ear" for the now defunct *Washington Star*.

(When the *Star* folded, she was hired by the *Post*, despite strong objections from some at the paper who thought her style of journalism beneath the dignity of a national newspaper. Her tour there ended not long after she falsley accused President Carter of bugging President-elect Reagan. She now writes her gossip column for the *Washington Times*.)

In 1978, "The Ear" was reputed to be the most widely read column in Washington, a claim that I do not question, and that says a great deal about our nation's capital. Though, to be fair, most public officials read it to make sure that they were not among that day's victims.

Because of the *Star*'s perilous financial position and the wide readership of the column, it was subjected to a minimum of editorial control. No editor of a paper that is losing millions each year wants to risk losing his most popular columnist. Even responsible reporters sometimes defended the excesses of "The Ear" because "it's helping to keep the *Star* alive."

Ms. McClellan had taken swipes at the President's daughter before, but on this particular morning she opened her column with a story depicting Amy as a spoiled brat who used her residence in the White House to get anything she wanted. At the time Amy was ten years old.

According to "The Ear," Amy's relay team had lost a race against another local elementary school. That part was true, but it was the only part.

She went on to claim that Amy "sat on the ground and howled . . . 'I want a trophy.'" At which point, a Secret Service agent "sneaked the sparkly gilt first-place trophy away in his jacket [and] gave it to the First Daughter." The real winners supposedly had to make do with the second-place trophy. The coach of the winning team then called them aside and threatened to throw anyone off the track team who breathed a word about the incident.

The whole thing was absurd; even if Amy had been the kind of child who pitched a temper tantrum over losing a race, which she decidedly was not, it is impossible to imagine a teacher and a Secret Service agent becoming involved in such foolishness.

As usual, Ms. McClellan had written her column without making any attempt to check with the people whose names she was defaming. Nor was she about to admit an error. Statements from school officials and Secret Service agents who had been at the event to the effect that nothing of the kind had occurred had no impact on her (which is not surprising), or on the editors of the *Star* (which is).

Ms. McClellan's response was simply to note in a subsequent column that her vicious little story had been denied, restate her contention that it was nevertheless true, and look for another chance to vent her spleen on Amy. Several months later she found it, and reported in her column that Amy had been disappointed when a shop did not have the item she was looking for. "The Ear" was glad to report "that she did not cry . . . but she did stamp one little foot."

The other thing that bothered me and others in the White House about press coverage of Amy was the pictures. I fully realize how subjective a subject that is. The tendency to read malice into an unflattering news photograph is almost reflexive among those in public life—even those who know better.

Still, it is a fact of life that the choosing of pictures can have a powerful effect on the impact of a story and on public perceptions of the person involved. It is also a fact that pictures tend to be chosen not only to convey the mood of a story, or because they are newsworthy in themselves, but because they conform to preexisting notions about the subject.

In Amy's case the preexisting notion was of a spoiled, not very happy, and singularly gawky and unattractive child. None of that fit the real Amy, except that she was in the White House at the time when she was going through those delightfully awkward and bittersweet years of transition from little girl to young woman. There were the glasses and braces, and a certain clumsy shyness with adults. She was in those years a surprisingly typical adolescent.

It started, I think, on her first day of school in Washington. Her mother took her down, as mothers are wont to do on such occasions. The press, of course, covered it as though it were the arrival in court of a Mafia don. There was, as might have been expected, precious little to write about. But there were the pictures.

The one that was chosen to run over most of the country showed Amy with eyes down and head ducked walking into the school building. The impression was of a terribly self-conscious little girl on the verge of tears because she had to go to school. The fact was that there was ice on the sidewalk and her downcast eyes and serious expression were the result of a desire not to lose her footing.

From that day forward, I can hardly remember any news photo of Amy that was not unflattering. There is certainly no rule that requires the news organizations to run only flattering photos of anyone. But it is widely understood to be an unwritten rule that unflattering photos of public officials are usually discarded. It always seemed to me that a child might have been due the same consideration that is accorded to fully grown men and women in statehouses and city halls across the land.

Journalists who are willing to defend the way their colleagues treated Amy, and to the credit of the institution they are few in number, claim that Amy's parents were responsible for the journalistic excesses. "After all," they say, "Amy was allowed to travel with the President and First Lady, and even to attend a state dinner—where, horror of horrors, she was observed reading a book."

One may agree or not with other parents' methods of raising their children. My own experience has been that nothing makes you humbler on the subject than trying to raise one of your own. However, I did not, and do not now, see anything wrong with allowing a child to experience some sense of the historic and important events going on around her—so long as the effort does not disrupt the business of government or unduly burden the taxpayers.

Amy was on all these occasions, so far as I was able to observe, an inoffensive and inexpensive spectator. She certainly never got drunk and made an ass of herself, which is more than one can say for some of those who took such exception to her presence.

As for reading the book at the state dinner, it seemed to me to be a remarkably constructive use of the time spent at such occasions.

AMARETTO
AND CREAM_____

Less than two months after publication of the "pyramids" story, the gossip side of the *Washington Post* struck again. That February of 1978, the *Washington Post Sunday Magazine* carried the most damaging accusation yet: Hamilton had supposedly spat a drink on a woman in Sarsfield's, a well-known Washington bar. It was damaging because of the nature of the accusation (it is difficult to imagine more disgusting behavior) and because I badly mishandled the response.

I first learned of what would become the "amaretto and cream" story on Thursday, February 16, prior to Sunday publication. An acquaintance called to say that reporters were "snooping around the bar on a story about Hamilton," but he had no details. A few hours later, a friend at the *Washington Post*, who still wishes to remain anonymous, called to describe a story by gossip columnist Rudy Maxa that would appear in that Sunday's *Post Magazine*.

Because the *Magazine* goes to press several days in advance, she had already seen the printed story. She was upset because the accusation sounded outrageous, and because the story contained no denial or comment from anyone at the White House. I asked if she could obtain a copy of the story for me, which she did— delivering it to a member of the press office staff that evening.

The story was waiting for me Friday morning when I arrived at the White House. I thought it was just about the trashiest piece of journalism I had ever seen.

Stretching halfway across the top of the page was a cartoon drawing of a disheveled and apparently intoxicated Hamilton Jordan with a drink dribbling down his face. Maxa's story ran below.

Hamilton had supposedly made suggestive remarks to a young woman while standing at the bar at Sarsfield's. According to Maxa, the woman was not interested, and Hamilton responded by spitting a mouthful of his drink down the front of her dress, not once, but twice. The story also contained an apparently unrelated item in which a young woman from California accused Hamilton of "grabbing" her several months earlier while they were dancing at a Los Angeles night spot.

(As it turned out, the apparently unrelated California story came from an old friend of the woman Hamilton had supposedly spat upon. She had "happened to call" while Maxa was working on the Scarfield story.)

The story was absurd. No one who knew Hamilton could imagine him doing anything so atrocious. After checking with Ham to see if Maxa had called him before the story was written (he had not), I called Maxa. I was told that he had left town and could not be reached. I explained my problem and demanded that they find some way to reach him. I also called Howard Simons, the managing editor of the *Post*, but was told that he, along with other *Post* executives, was at an annual retreat and seminar.

It was obviously too late to get a denial run with the story. A conversation with Maxa would be useful only if I could learn anything from him that would help me prepare a response.

Reporters are quite good at writing around the weak spots in their stories. Those who deal in gossip are better than most. Comments or statements that tend to cast doubt on the allegation being made tend to get left in the reporter's notebook. But most of them cannot resist the temptation to defend what they have written when it is challenged. In the process, they often unintentionally reveal contradictions or inadequate research. Even getting mad is helpful. If the reporter also becomes angry, the chances that he or she will say something interesting are increased.

Later that day, Maxa called back. He had not been out of town, just away from his desk. He was upset that I had a copy of the story, and demanded to know how I got it. I was even more angry, and the conversation was heated. I made some pointed and unflattering comments about people who make their living "ruining lives and reputations with concocted garbage" and asked why we had not been given a chance to at least deny the story.

Maxa said he had no trouble sleeping at night and that he had spoken with a secretary in the press office, but no one had gotten back to him. I countered that getting a comment on something this important might have been worth more than one dime.

Maxa said that the young woman involved in the incident had called him with the story. He said she had two witnesses, a girlfriend who had gone with her to the bar and a man they met after they got there. He placed particular emphasis on the man's confirmation of the story, since he was supposedly unbiased, having met the two women for the first time that evening. (I later discovered that this "unbiased" source knew both of the women well. He would not talk to me about the incident because he was married and did not want his wife to know he frequented singles bars.)

I asked if he had interviewed the bartender, since bartenders are usually considered the ultimate judge of barroom disputes. He said he had not because the woman involved told him that he "was at the other end of the bar and did not see any of what happened."

As I reviewed my notes, several points seemed to be interesting. For example, it seemed unlikely that there would have been only one bartender working the entire length of the bar on a Friday night in such a popular establishment.

I decided to try to find the one who had been closest to see what he had to say. My suspicions about Maxa's motives and about how much confidence he had in his own story, which had been aroused by his cursory attempt to obtain a White House reaction, were increased by his failure to make any effort to see if the bartender had witnessed the incident.

By the afternoon of the next day, we had located the bartender, a young man named Danny Marshall. He had seen the incident and was willing to speak on the record about it. He told a story that flatly contradicted Maxa's column.

He said it had all taken place right in front of him. Hamilton was seated directly across the bar from his drink station, and on a busy night, such as the one in question, he never moved more than two or three steps from that position. The women, who had been drinking vodka to the point that he was worried about their walking away without paying their check, approached Hamilton. They had already "had too much to drink," had become "obnoxious," and had "spilled a couple of drinks."

There was, he said, "an exchange of words." He did not hear

what was said and could not say who was at fault, but he was certain that there had been no spitting. He said that he then presented the women with a check and asked them to leave. They became indignant and abusive, declaring that "nobody can talk to me that way" and threatening to "go to the newspapers."

He said that neither of the women in their protests to him about being asked to leave had said anything about being spat upon. Nor did their dresses show evidence of spitting. There were a number of regular customers standing nearby who "had their eye on Hamilton because they knew who he was," and none of them came up to Marshall at the time or later to say, "Hey, did you see him spit on . . . this girl."

The bartender's statement seemed to be a godsend. Now we had one of the bastards dead to rights. I was more than relieved, almost jubilant. We could not only disprove and discredit this bit of libel, but in the process cast doubt on similar stories, including Sally Quinn's pyramids item. Perhaps we could even provoke a hard look by serious journalists at this whole business of gossip mongering.

I had underreacted to the pyramids story. The simple denial had been dismissed as routine. Most of Washington had been left with the impression that the allegations were true and Hamilton ran into questions about it almost everywhere he went. I was determined not to make the same mistake again. I did not. I made exactly the opposite mistake, with even more disastrous consequences.

I called Mike Cardozo, deputy to the White House counsel, and asked him to go out and interview Marshall, record the answers, and give me the transcript. In the meantime, I dictated an account of my conversation with Maxa, pointing out weaknesses and inconsistencies in his reporting on the story. I also asked two of Hamilton's friends who had been with him that night to put their recollections in writing.

My idea was to collect all the evidence, present it to the flock of reporters who would soon be asking for our response to the allegations, and let them make their own judgment.

Once the story actually appeared on Sunday, the wire services began to clatter out their rewrites. That night, the *CBS Evening News* relayed the *Post*'s accusations to several million people.

On Monday morning I released the statements contradicting Maxa's charges. The reporters made their own judgments all right, but not about Rudy Maxa or the accuracy of his allegations.

Their reaction was predictable, but unfortunately I had failed to predict it. The stories that night and the next day concentrated not on the holes in Maxa's story or on the bartender's refutation of it, but on the number of pages in the statement we handed out.

"White House issues thirty-three-page document to defend Jordan" (or twenty-two- or twenty-four-page, depending on which reporter was doing the counting) was the theme of the stories. My overreaction became the issue rather than the accuracy of the accusations.

It was a painful and bitter lesson for me. The results for Hamilton were even worse. With a new angle to pursue, the press gave extensive and prolonged coverage to the charges. Editorial comment and cartoons, almost all negative and some of them vicious, flowed into the news summary office for three weeks.

The *Boston Globe* decided that Hamilton had "deserved what he got," although no one at the *Globe* had made any effort to follow up on Maxa's story. The *Globe* also cavalierly informed its readers that Hamilton had a drinking problem (which was untrue) but neglected to provide any basis for the allegation.

Although its Washington bureau chief had described the Maxa story as "junk journalism," the *New York Daily News* took the President to task for "yanking a staffer off official duties to find evidence disputing" the Maxa story—conveniently ignoring the fact that the interview with Danny Marshall had taken place on a Saturday.

Haynes Johnson, a usually thoughtful columnist and writer at the *Post*, appeared on the *Today* show to denounce the waste of time in responding to the charges, while stoutly maintaining that there was nothing wasteful or improper in the *Post*'s developing and publishing such allegations.

This reaction from the *Post* and the *Daily News* displayed the arrogance and defensiveness of the fourth estate at its worst. It is apparently all right for journalists to publish unsubstantiated or questionable allegations against a public official even though the charges are bound to impair his ability to do his job, as well as damage his personal reputation. But heaven forbid that the victim's friends and colleagues should devote any of their time to establishing his innocence.

This type of reaction is also typical of the double standard that journalists so lovingly nurture: defend and make excuses for the most questionable behavior by a fellow journalist while seeking every opportunity to condemn and discredit any attempt to defend the victim of such shoddy practices.

Syndicated columnist Ellen Goodman decided on the basis of her experience with recently divorced men that the allegations against Hamilton "had the ring of truth to them." Neither she nor most of the other commentators had found the time to read the statements issued in his defense.

In the midst of the reaction to all of this, Hamilton's father died. As he was walking through Washington's National Airport on his way to the funeral, Hamilton was accosted by a young man who loudly berated him about the Maxa and Quinn stories all the way to the gate. Afraid of what would be written if he was involved in a public incident, Hamilton ducked his head without responding and tried to ignore his tormentor.

Looking back on all three of the early stories involving Hamilton, and with the benefit of hours of interviews with the reporters and witnesses involved, I think several points are worth making.

I should begin by saying that I am even more convinced now than I was at the time that the accusations against Hamilton were false. The reader has a right to know that up front. I hope I will be believed when I say that if I had come to a different conclusion, I would have said so.

The most obvious conclusion that can be drawn is that I reacted poorly to both the Quinn and the Maxa stories. Had I taken the time to identify and call the people who sat at the table with Hamilton and Mrs. Ghorbal, I would have discovered a number of interesting things. The most important is that there is by any reasonable standard considerable doubt about what happened that night.

Syndicated columnist Art Buchwald says, "That story was crap. I was sitting there, and it didn't happen."

Helen Strauss, wife of former Democratic party Chairman

Robert Strauss, agrees, although her language is a bit more delicate.

Henry Kissinger, who was seated on Mrs. Ghorbal's right, says he did not hear the pyramids remark or see Hamilton pluck at anyone's dress.

Mrs. Simcha Dinitz, wife of the Israeli ambassador, was seated on Hamilton's left. She is sure that "nothing improper took place."

And Mrs. Ghorbal herself says flatly that Hamilton neither did nor said anything impolite in her presence.

ABC White House correspondent Sam Donaldson, who was seated across the table from Hamilton and Mrs. Ghorbal, is the one person at the table who says he heard what was described in the Quinn story. Although he says he did not see Hamilton touch Mrs. Ghorbal or her dress, he is sure that he heard him make the comment about wanting to see the pyramids.

Mrs. Dinitz says she remembers a totally innocent conversation between Hamilton and Henry Kissinger in which pyramids were mentioned, and suggests that it might have been misinterpreted by someone who did not hear it clearly.

A person at another table says Hamilton did make a comment about Mrs. Ghorbal's bosom, not to her, but in a joking and slightly inebriated conversation involving Hamilton, himself, and Donaldson after everyone had gotten up from dinner.

Donaldson feels certain that he did not misunderstand and that the comment was made at the table, to Mrs. Ghorbal.

While I was researching the amaretto and cream story for this book, a new bit of information came to light, interesting enough to merit an extra round of interviews. I had been discussing our heated telephone conversation of two years prior with Rudy Maxa, when he stated that a friend of his had heard Hamilton admit that the spitting story was true.

According to Maxa, this friend spent an evening with Hamilton and a number of other people not long after the story appeared. In the course of that evening, he asked Hamilton if the story was accurate, and Hamilton responded, "Yes, but Maxa didn't have to write it."

I asked Maxa why he had never written about this confirmation, since we had been loudly and publicly denying his story. He said he "just didn't see any need in dredging it all up again."

Maxa's friend was David Burgin, then a sports editor for the *Washington Star* and now editor of the *Orlando Sentinel*. He remembers the night in question, and he remembers telling Maxa about it, but his recollections differ from Maxa's in two respects.

Burgin says Hamilton never said, "Yes [it's true], but Maxa didn't have to write it," or anything else that explicitly confirmed the story. Nor, says Burgin, did he ever tell Maxa that Hamilton had made such a statement. What Burgin says he told Maxa was that there was a great deal of joking and kidding around about the story on that evening and that he "got the impression from all that was said that the story was true."

Burgin also says that when Maxa talked to him, he was eager to use the incident in his column. The reason he did not, according to Burgin, was that Burgin refused permission, saying that it had taken place in his house and he thought such use would be improper.

There is reason to believe that Maxa did try to get confirmation of this "confession," but was not able to find it. A bureau chief for a large daily paper who was present that evening remembers Maxa calling him shortly after the night in question asking about what had happened.

Even more to the point, this reporter remembers the conversation about the spitting incident, and he came away from it with an impression exactly the opposite of Burgin's.

"My reaction," he says, "was that there had been some sort of an incident, but that spitting was not a part of it. I certainly would have remembered if Hamilton had said, 'Yes, I spit a drink on that woman,' or anything like that."

Three others, who were present that night, all agree that there was talk about the incident "in a spirit of drunken levity," as one put it. "People were trying to kid Hamilton out of taking the thing so hard. There were comments like 'Try to keep that one in your glass,' and 'Be nice to this guy or he'll spit on you.'"

But they all say that they heard nothing that tended to confirm the story. One, who is a friend of Hamilton's, says:

"Everyone had been drinking and none of us may be good

witnesses; but if Ham had said anything that even implied that he had done that, I know I would have remembered. I had been telling everyone all over Washington that the thing wasn't so. To hear Hamilton say that it was, particularly in front of people that neither of us knew very well, is not something I would forget."

It is interesting that two reporters participating in the same conversation—Burgin and the bureau chief—came away with totally contradictory impressions of what was said. Furthermore, Burgin and Maxa have significantly differing recollections of what they said to each other.

Even if Maxa's original story had been true, it makes no sense that Hamilton would have casually confirmed it to a group of his friends who had been vigorously defending him publicly and privately for the past several weeks, because of his personal assurances that the story was untrue. That he would refute himself in front of other people he hardly knew, some of whom he had only met for the first time that night, is even more difficult to accept.

Nor does it make sense that others at Burgin's house, including those who are Hamilton's friends, would still be lying to protect him. They are also my friends, and some are also friends and close supporters of the President's. What they supposedly heard that night would have been confirmation that Hamilton had been lying to all of us, including the President—something they would never have tolerated.

In Burgin's case, I do not doubt that he came away from the evening with the impression that he relates. I suspect that it was less definite than he claims even now, and that his refusal to let Maxa write about it had something to do with his standards of accuracy as well as his concern for the privacy of his home.

The bottom line, as people in Washington used to say, is the behavior of Maxa himself. His last-minute attempt to substantiate his allegation turned out to be almost as sloppy and implausible as the original column. The gentleman has either a very bad memory or little regard for the truth.

STUDIO 54: TRAVESTY AND TRAGEDY

Having established the atmosphere that existed by the late summer of 1979 and learned something about how it came to be that way, we may now turn to the way the press handled the allegations that Hamilton Jordan had used cocaine in a New York disco called Studio 54. What follows is an account of a personal tragedy with national implications. It involves the ethics of journalists and lawyers, the judgment of government officials, and even the equity of the law.

Even four years after it all occurred, as I write about and relive those days, anger, frustration, and bitterness come flooding back. Justice was not done. The innocent suffered more than the guilty. And some of the guilty paid no price at all. The chance for redress, except in the court of public opinion, has passed. If there is any good reason for telling this story now, it is the hope that an understanding of how such an injustice occurred will help to keep such a thing from happening again. I wish I could believe that it would.

In August of 1979, President Carter decided to spend his summer vacation aboard the riverboat *Delta Queen*, cruising the Mississippi River from Minneapolis to St. Louis. A few months earlier, on June 28, Ian Schrager and Steve Rubell had been indicted by a federal grand jury for tax fraud, conspiracy, and obstruction of justice. Rubell and Schrager were the owners of

Studio 54, a tacky-trendy nightclub in New York that catered to the exhibitionistic tendencies of the would-be beautiful people. One of the attractions of the night spot was the availability of a variety of drugs on the house for selected patrons.

As President Carter was preparing to leave for his vacation, Rubell and Schrager and their lawyers, Roy Cohn and Mitchell Rogovin, set in motion a plan to circumvent the penalties of the law. They would charge that the chief of staff to the President had used cocaine at Studio 54 and attempt to use that information to pressure the Justice Department into agreeing to reduced sentences.

Their plan failed, partially because of the ineptitude of the lawyers. Hamilton Jordan was eventually cleared. Steve Rubell and Ian Schrager went to jail for tax fraud. But the attempt to make it work almost ruined the public career of the President's senior aide. He was left with staggering legal bills and permanent damage to his reputation. It eroded the credibility of a President and set the stage for behavior by journalists and lawyers that called into question their judgment and their integrity.

As the President was ending his cruise, Mr. Rogovin presented the Justice Department with his accusation. On an evening in April of 1978, Rogovin said, Hamilton Jordan had come to Studio 54. While there, he had asked for and been given cocaine in the presence of Jody Powell, Steve Rubell, and a small-time drug dealer called Johnny C.

As required by the Ethics in Government Act, the Attorney General directed the FBI to investigate immediately.

When the *Delta Queen* reached Lock and Dam Number 24, near the town of Clarksville, Missouri, shortly after 7 P.M. on Thursday, August 23, 1979, President Carter was summoned to the lockmaster's office, where a scrambler phone had been installed. The Attorney General wanted to talk to him, and he wanted to talk on a secure line.

As the senior staff member on the trip, I walked the few dozen yards with the President, and was standing beside him as he took the call. After less than a minute of conversation, which came mostly from the other end of the line, the President interrupted to say that I was in the room. A few seconds later, he motioned for me to step outside. I thought the call must involve some sensitive intelligence matter about which I had no need to know, and was curious but not concerned.

Once back on board, I asked the President if he could tell me anything about the call, since the press had seen him break away from the crowd and go into the lockmaster's office. He said no. In a few minutes, one of the reporters in the small press pool aboard the *Delta Queen* asked why the President had gone to the office. I said that he had taken a phone call, but that I could not say anything more about it.

I dismissed the incident from my mind until several hours later, when the *Delta Queen* got under way from Lock 25 at Winfield, Missouri. The President asked if anyone had come on board to talk to me. Somewhat puzzled, I said no. He said FBI agents would probably be waiting at the next lock to ask me some questions. There was nothing more that he could tell me, not even the reason for the questions. I was not to discuss what little I knew with anyone before talking with the FBI, and I was to cooperate with them completely.

At almost the same moment, FBI agents were arriving at Hamilton Jordan's apartment in northwest Washington to confront him with Rogovin's accusations. He had been called a few hours earlier, and quickly agreed to see the agents that night.

Although I knew nothing about that event, I was beginning to think the situation was a little strange. It would be four o'clock in the morning when we arrived at the next stop. Less than six hours later we would be in St. Louis, where the agents were most certainly based.

I had become accustomed to strange happenings over the past few years; some eventually made sense and others still do not. Even FBI interviews were not particularly startling occurrences. I had been through them before. But this appeared to be different. Why the haste, and why was the President able to tell me so little about what was going on? From the little I knew about FBI procedures, it almost looked as though I were the target of the investigation. I was almost right.

At four-fifteen on Friday morning we reached Lock and Dam 26 near Alton, Illinois. I stood along the lower deck railing watching for people who looked like FBI agents, and hoping they would spot me if I did not see them. I had told our advance people that there might be someone waiting to see me at this stop (although in accordance with the President's instructions, I did not say who). I had informed the Secret Service that some people from the FBI would be coming to talk to me, since the Secret Service would have to know who they were and why they were there to clear them on board. By that time, my feelings were about equally divided between concern and curiosity.

Shortly after four-thirty, a Secret Service agent brought two men up the gangway and introduced them as "the people who wanted to talk to you." The agents presented identification, apologized for the late hour, and asked if I was too tired to talk; they could wait until I got some sleep and see me in the morning. At that point, concern pulled ahead of curiosity. The last thing I wanted to do was wait until morning. The thought also occurred to me that if a serious problem was developing, I would have the rest of the night to think about how to handle it. They asked if there was a place where we could sit and speak privately, and I took them into the cabin-deck lounge nearby.

The lounge had long been deserted for the night and the lights turned out. After a brief and unsuccessful search for a light switch, we sat at a table near a window illuminated by the giant floodlights along the lock and the glare of television lights following the President as he shook hands with the several hundred people who had driven out to greet him. Their cheers and applause as he moved along drifted through the open windows.

The senior agent quickly relieved some of my concern by telling me that I was not the target of their investigation. He then asked if I was familiar with or had ever visited a place called Studio 54 in New York. I told him I had never been to Studio 54, and, from what I knew of it, thought I was probably not their kind of people. He said, with only a trace of a smile and a raised eyebrow toward his partner, that it might be a short session in that case, and outlined the allegations.

I said that to the best of my recollection (which turned out to be accurate), Hamilton Jordan and I had never been in New York on the same night in all of 1978. He then asked if I was familiar with about half a dozen names. I was not, but I, and most of the rest of the country, very shortly would be. After about thirty minutes, they thanked me for my time, apologized again for the inconvenient hour, and left.

A few hours earlier in Washington, after waiving his right to have an attorney present, Hamilton flatly denied that he had ever used cocaine, at Studio 54 or anywhere else. He said he had somewhat reluctantly made one, relatively brief, visit to Studio 54, but had not even been in New York during April of 1978, when the incident had allegedly taken place.

As we pulled away from Alton, I told the President about the interview and what I had said to the FBI. He seemed somewhat relieved, but still concerned. So was I.

Neither of us believed there was any truth to the charges. We both knew of Hamilton's strong distaste for the drug scene. I had heard him warn young staffers of the risk to their careers if they were foolish enough to indulge in it. I had volunteered to the FBI that I had never seen or even heard of Hamilton's ever using drugs, and could not believe that he had done so.

But we both knew that innocence is not necessarily a defense. We had seen the tremendous momentum that can build behind an allegation of scandal against a public official.

Soon after I became involved in politics and press work, an older and more experienced hand had warned that it only takes about five seconds for someone to call you an SOB, but proving that you are not one can take a bit longer. That would be the crux of the problem. It would take nine months.

The press has never been known for adhering to particularly strict rules of evidence, or fair play, when dealing with stories of scandal in high places. There is no concept of innocent until proven guilty; there is no right to confront, much less cross examine, your accuser. Too often, there is little or no restraint on the publication of the rankest sort of hearsay and innuendo. That is bad enough. Now, however, the problem was exacerbated by the law itself.

The new Ethics in Government Act, which had become law the year before, contained a provision that required the Attorney General to investigate thoroughly any charge of criminal behavior made against any person on a list of 140 government officials, no matter how frivolous the accusation or how incredible its source. If the investigation did not, within ninety days, show the charge to be without substance (if, in effect, the Justice Department was not able to prove that the accused was innocent), the Attorney General had to appoint a special prosecutor.

The Carter administration, although favoring the act in general, had opposed that provision. We would soon have reason to wish we had been much more vigorous in our opposition.

To protect the reputation of those falsely accused, the act required that the preliminary investigation and the appointment of a special prosecutor be kept confidential. But the drafters of the law had reckoned without the likes of Schrager and Rubell and their two lawyers, Rogovin and Cohn. They were quite a quartet.

Mitchell Rogovin was a well-known Washington insider with extensive political and press connections; Roy Cohn was equally well connected in New York. Both had experience in government, Rogovin as counsel to the IRS and the CIA during the Nixon and Ford administrations, and Cohn as a chief aide to Senator Joseph McCarthy in the fifties.

Both certainly knew that if an allegation as flimsy as the one made against Jordan was brought directly to a responsible news organization, the allegation might never be publicized. An allegation is by definition conjectural. It may or may not be true. Before publishing an allegation, good news operations will usually make some attempt to check it out, to see if there is anything to it.

But an FBI investigation of a high government official had always been considered in a different light. The allegation under investigation might or might not be true, but the FBI investigation itself is a fact. The unwritten rule had been: "If the FBI thinks there is enough substance to launch an investigation, there is enough substance for us to run the story."

The Ethics in Government Act had changed the rules for the FBI. An investigation under this law did not in any way imply a judgment by the FBI on the substantiation of the accusation. Unfortunately for Hamilton Jordan and for the Carter administration, it quickly became apparent that no matter how the rules had changed for the FBI, the rules of press behavior remained the same. The existence of an investigation would continue to be sufficient rationale for extensive coverage.

At about 9 A.M. on Friday morning when the *Delta Queen* reached St. Louis, a few hours after my session with the FBI, I called Hamilton. We agreed that we faced a serious problem. But we had no inkling of just how serious it would be.

There had been other investigations under the Ethics in Government Act that had remained confidential as the law required, so we had some hope that this one would be handled quickly and without inflammatory press coverage. Nevertheless, we decided that press calls would probably come sooner or later. Fortunately, we decided that we had better be prepared for sooner.

By two that afternoon, I was back in the White House. Hamilton had already received a call from the *New York Times*. They had been told that the FBI was investigating drug charges against him. What did he have to say for himself?

The *Times* had learned of the accusations on August 22, two days before Hamilton knew anything about them.

As it turned out, the *Times* also scooped both the Attorney General and the FBI. Attorney General Benjamin Civiletti received his first briefing on the charges, which had first been raised with the U.S. attorney for the Southern District of New York, late in the afternoon of August 23. He and senior Justice Department officials quickly concluded that an investigation was required under the Ethics in Government Act, and it should begin immediately.

The interviews would be more effective if they were conducted cold—without advance warning to either Hamilton or me. The officials were concerned, with justification as it turned out, that the press might get hold of the allegations. Publicity could give the two suspects a chance to compare notes. The Department of Justice also wanted to make sure it was clear that an investigation had begun without prodding by the press. The best way to do that was to make sure it was under way before the first story ran.

Attorney General Civiletti placed a call to William Webster, the director of the FBI. He was out of town and could not be reached immediately. Calls were placed to Webster's immediate subordinates, Homer Boynton and Francis M. Mullen, Jr., executive assistant directors of the FBI. By this time, the sun was going down and both men had left the bureau. They were quickly located and told to report to the Attorney General's office immediately. In the meantime, Webster was contacted in South Dakota. Since the conversation was over a standard telephone line, Civiletti gave the FBI director only a general description of the situation. Arrangements were made for a more detailed briefing by secure channels.

Within an hour, Boynton and Mullen arrived at the Justice Department. Both were in shirt sleeves. Boynton had been in the middle of a swim and came in with his longish, curly hair still wet.

By the time they arrived, Terry (Terrence B.) Adamson, special assistant to the Attorney General and director of public information for the Justice Department, had determined that Hamilton was in town and should be at home that night. He had also pulled the schedule for the *Delta Queen* so that plans could be made for contacting the President on a secure phone line and placing FBI agents on board to interrogate me.

Boynton and Mullen were briefed by Bob Fiske, the U.S. attorney for the Southern District of New York. He was responsible for the prosecution of the tax evasion charges against Rubell and Schrager, and the charges against Hamilton had been made to him by Rogovin, Schrager's attorney. Rogovin had been hinting to Fiske that he had information about wrongdoing by a high government official for several days, but he had not detailed the charges or mentioned Hamilton Jordan's name until the day before, August 22.

Arrangements were made to brief the agents who would conduct the interrogations. The Attorney General picked up the red scrambler phone on his desk and asked the operator to connect him with the President as soon as possible. Civiletti, who had just become Attorney General a week earlier following the resignation of Griffin Bell, had the unenviable responsibility of telling the President that two members of his senior staff were implicated in a drug investigation. Civiletti knew that if the charges were true, both Hamilton and I would have to resign. He also knew that even if they were false, we and the President were in for some difficult days. Looking back on it now, he says he had no idea how difficult.

When I got back to the White House on Friday afternoon, the first person I saw was neither the President nor Hamilton. My wife had come down to meet me. I had been gone for over a week, and since the President had no scheduled activities for the rest of the day, we were looking forward to an early start on the weekend. I had only a few minutes to prepare her for what was coming. I closed the door to my office and told her what had happened, trying to be as reassuring as I could.

I told her I felt certain I could eventually prove that I had never been to Studio 54, but the job of proving Hamilton had not used drugs would be more difficult. Still, I thought we would come out all right in the end. I did not try to be overly optimistic. I had learned long ago that Nan would not pry or push me to talk about things I did not want to discuss; but she preferred the truth with the bark off—the worst-case possibilities up front rather than nasty surprises later on.

I also told her that there would soon be press coverage and that my name was likely to be prominently mentioned in the early stories. I asked her to call our twelve-year-old daughter, Emily, and tell her what was happening. Emily was visiting my mother in Vienna, Georgia, so Nan could explain it all to my mother, too. My mother would then tell my aunt, who lives on the adjacent farm. Between them, they would make sure that hometown friends and family were adequately briefed.

This process of calling Vienna to warn of and explain some impending difficulty had become routine. I sometimes thought that Washington gossips could have gleaned better material at Ruth Pennington's beauty parlor in Vienna than at all the Washington cocktail parties they attended. Their coiffures and their livers would also have benefited.

I could not tell whether the glint in Nan's eyes was anger or tears—perhaps both.

"They're trying to destroy Hamilton," she said. "This thing will just drag on and on. They're lying, and everyone knows they're lying, but that won't matter. Ham is going to be hurt, and you and the President. But nothing will ever happen to the people responsible for all this."

She and I both knew that she was probably right. I could not think of anything to say. Nan gave me a smile and a hug and left.

As she left to drive back home, I walked around the corner to join Hamilton in the Oval Office. We reviewed the situation with the President, including the fact that the *New York Times* was already working on the story. I said that I was not sure yet, but thought we would be better off talking to the *Times*. Perhaps we could get them to hold off for a day or two. If not, we would at least get our side into the first story.

The President said he was inclined to agree, but to handle it as we saw fit. He seldom became involved in the details of press relations. Usually, as in this case, it made my job easier. At other times I wished that he would take a greater interest in the nuances of the relationship.

Although I did not know it until later, Hamilton had slipped back into the Oval Office to offer his resignation. He was profoundly upset and discouraged. He argued that even though he was innocent, it would take a long time to prove it. In the meantime, the adverse publicity and the distraction from the other issues were too much of a burden for the President to bear.

The President would have none of it. He refused to accept the resignation and encouraged Hamilton to fight it out. If he resigned, the President said, we would have the worst of both worlds: Hamilton's services would be lost, and the resignation would be taken as an admission of guilt. Hamilton agreed to stay on, but he would come close to submitting his resignation more than once during the next nine months.

Once Hamilton and I had reviewed our notes, I was convinced that we should invite the *New York Times* people over for a talk. We had a good story to tell. The allegation was demonstrably inaccurate in three major respects:

- The incident was supposed to have taken place in April, but Hamilton's logs would show that he had not spent a night in New York during that month.

- Our daily schedules would show that Hamilton and I had not spent the same night in New York during the entire year.

- I was supposed to have been with Hamilton, but I had never been to Studio 54 in my life.

Hamilton was concerned that talking to the press might create problems for him with the Justice Department. He knew that the law required that the investigation be kept secret. He did not want officials at Justice or the FBI to think he was attempting to short-circuit their efforts by taking his case to the press. I argued that if the *Times* had been told enough to have a story anyway, no one could fault us for responding to their questions. I thought, but did not say, that there was little chance the stories would be favorable enough to Hamilton to place any pressure on Justice to bend in his direction.

To resolve the issue, I called Bill Kovach, the new Washington editor of the *Times*, and asked him to tell me what they had. After listening to his description, there was no doubt in my mind that they had enough for a story, no matter what we did. I told him that the whole thing was a crock of shit, but that I would have to do some checking on just what more Hamilton and I could say and get right back to him.

Kovach and I both knew that the deadline for the edition of the *Times* that is delivered to homes in Washington is 6:00 P.M. He wanted to make that edition with what was definitely a "Washington story." I wanted to make sure that we had plenty of time to point out the errors and inconsistencies in the allegations. I also hoped that we might be able to cast enough doubt on the credibility of the charges to get the *Times* to hold the story for a day or two. That would give us time to try to come up with other witnesses or information that would support Hamilton's innocence—and mine.

Next, I called Terry Adamson. Terry was uniquely qualified to be the Attorney General's spokesman. He was a lawyer who had worked as a reporter. He and I had developed a good relationship, keeping each other posted on developing matters that might become issues in the press. The purpose of this call was to make sure he knew that the *New York Times* was working on the Studio 54 story and to ask whether he thought anyone at Justice would think it improper for Hamilton and me to talk to the *Times*.

Adamson said he had already received an inquiry from the *Times*, but had made no comment, as the law required. However, he saw no problem at Justice if Hamilton and I wanted to present our side of the story. If we decided to do that, Adamson said, it might make sense for the Justice Department to release a short statement confirming that the investigation was under way.

With Hamilton's agreement, I called Kovach and asked if he could come to the White House and see us. Since neither Kovach nor I had any interest in other news organizations' finding out about the story, I told him we would meet in Hamilton's office rather than mine, which was often surrounded by reporters. I would also arrange for him to enter through the West Lobby rather than the press room.

The *New York Times* bureau is located at the corner of Connecticut Avenue and K Street, less than four blocks from the White House. Kovach said he would see us in fifteen minutes, and was bringing Nicholas Horrock, their chief investigative reporter, and Phil Taubman, another investigative reporter who occasionally covered the Justice Department.

In the short time before they arrived, I tried to give Hamilton, who spent little time with the press, a quick briefing on the people who would be interrogating him.

Kovach had come to Washington only a couple of weeks before. I had done some calling around when his appointment as bureau chief was announced, and had made a point of asking him out for a get-acquainted drink as soon as he hit town. I was favorably impressed by what I saw and what I had heard about him. His reputation was that of a steady, nonflamboyant professional. His job would be to run the bureau. He would not write stories himself. That meant I no longer had to worry about being caught in the middle between the bureau chief and a White House correspondent when the correspondent felt that his territory was being invaded by his boss.

I liked his soft-spoken manner and his thoughtful approach to the job. On top of that, he was a southerner. I would not have to explain to him what "born again" meant, and when he had a few drinks too many, I would not have to sit and listen to mildly insulting imitations of the President's accent.

Horrock was a different matter. I had dealt with him only occasionally and had no major, specific complaints, but my general impression of him was not encouraging. He seemed to be almost a caricature of an investigative reporter: aggressive, suspicious of anyone in public office, and inclined to browbeat and intimidate when he thought he could get away with it. In addition, other reporters at the *Times* said he made no effort to hide his distaste for southerners in general, and those in the White House in particular. Finally, I had been warned that Horrock was determined that the *Times* would never again be beaten on a White

House scandal as it had been by the *Washington Post* during Watergate.

I had no strong impressions of Phil Taubman one way or the other. He had worked on several stories that involved the White House, and I remembered him as generally reasonable and not excessively prosecutorial.

Our approach would be to speak freely since there was nothing to hide, but to be careful not to say anything unless we were sure it was true. I had learned the hard way that there is little toleration for an honest mistake when talking with the press. We did have the advantage of dealing with only one newspaper and in a relatively informal setting. It is much easier to explain a complicated point or to persuade a reporter that you are telling the truth in that sort of situation than in the supercharged atmosphere of a White House briefing.

I also felt we were fortunate to be dealing with the *New York Times*. I considered the *Times* to be more careful, more thorough, and less given to hyperbole than most other news organizations. That opinion would become somewhat tarnished in the weeks to come.

There were no big surprises in the interview. Horrock did most of the questioning: "Did you use cocaine at Studio 54? Have you ever used cocaine? Have you ever been to Studio 54? Did anyone offer you drugs or to set you up with a piece of ass? Do you remember going to the basement [where the cocaine sniffing had allegedly taken place]?"

Hamilton denied that he had ever used cocaine, acknowledged that he had visited Studio 54, said he was not certain whether he had been in the basement, but felt sure he would remember if anyone had offered sex or drugs, and he did not.

I denied that I had ever been to Studio 54, and Hamilton confirmed that I had not been with him on the one occasion when he was there.

We both described our sessions with the FBI and stressed that we had cooperated fully and strictly abided by their request not to discuss the matter with those who had been with Hamilton that night until after the FBI had interviewed them.

I was mildly surprised that Hamilton was asked whether he had ever used cocaine. I knew, as did the reporter who asked the question, that drug use is not unknown among some reporters in the *New York Times* Washington bureau. Later, I would discover that an informal screening process had taken place at the *Times* to make sure that reporters who used drugs were not assigned to work on this story. (One Timesman explained to me that he had worked on stories with one *Times* reporter who was spending "several hundred dollars per week on drugs.")

I was glad that Hamilton was able to issue a sweeping denial. I thought it would lend credibility to his denial of the specific charge. I was wrong.

I also noted with interest that Horrock said the *Times* had been told that the incident took place "sometime during the spring of '78" rather than April of '78. This was somewhat disappointing, since "April of '78" was one of the provable inaccuracies in the story. At the same time, it was the first real clue as to who had given the story to the *Times*.

The FBI had specifically mentioned April to Hamilton and to me, so it was unlikely that the leak had come from the Justice Department. That was reassuring. We had enough on our plates without having to worry about whether someone in the FBI or at a high level at Justice was gunning for Hamilton or me.

It was logical to assume that if the source for the *Times* was not the Justice Department, it must have been the defendants in the tax evasion case or their lawyers. This seemed important because it meant that the *Times* was getting its information from a source with an ax to grind.

Furthermore, since Justice had gotten the April date from the person who made the allegation to them, it seemed possible that the source for the *New York Times* was someone else—not the person who was talking to Justice. Although this was interesting, I did not know what to make of it, except that our antagonists might not have taken the time to get their stories completely straight.

Once we had set out the facts to the best of our knowledge, I tried to convince the *Times* to wait for a day or two before running the story. They had not interviewed any one of the four or five people who had been with Hamilton at Studio 54, and I felt sure that when they did, their responses would support Hamilton's story. However, it quickly became obvious that I was fighting a losing battle. Kovach pointed out that if they knew about the story, other papers would soon be on to it. They were not going to risk losing their scoop. He also argued that they would handle it more responsibly than some others, so we would be better off if their story was the first. Although I did not say so, I knew he was right.

After the interview was completed, Hamilton went up to talk to Lloyd Cutler, the President's legal counsel. Cutler is an experienced and well-connected Washington hand. He would be an excellent source of advice, but it seemed apparent that Hamilton would need outside counsel. Cutler was the President's lawyer; for him to be the primary source of legal advice for Hamilton could create a conflict of interest. Though we did not know it at the time, the sheer volume of the work that would have to be done would also have made it impossible for Cutler to represent Hamilton and perform his White House duties.

I returned to the press office to set in motion the work that would need to be done to handle the flood of questions that would come when the story appeared the next day. I had briefed Deputy Press Secretary Rex Granum that morning in St. Louis. My secretary, Carolyn Shields, was already pulling all my travel records for 1978 so I could try to prove that I had never been to Studio 54. I gave Rex an update on the *Times* interview and told him to make sure we had adequate staff on Saturday to handle the work load. The President had left for Camp David, and normally the press office would have been manned by a skeleton staff over the weekend.

There was one additional problem. Rex pointed out that I had a potential conflict of interest. He was right, but I was so caught up in the problem that it had not crossed my mind. How could I be the spokesman for the White House on this matter when I was implicated in the charge? Although it seemed unlikely, the time could come when to say something would be in my best interest but not the President's, or vice versa. We decided that for the time being it would be best for Rex to issue any statements and respond to any questions on this issue. He would also try to explain my awkward situation to reporters.

I then called Terry Adamson in the Justice Department press office, with Rex on an extension, to fill him in on our interview with the *Times* and to let him know that Rex would serve as the official spokesman on this issue. This would simplify things for Adamson, too. He could carry on routine discussions about the story with the White House Press Office without worrying about the problem of talking directly to someone who was involved in the investigation.

Adamson said that the Attorney General had decided that the department would issue a brief statement confirming the existence of the investigation when the *Times* story appeared the next day. He promised to let Rex know exactly what the statement would say as soon as it had been cleared.

The story in the *Times* the next day was about what we had expected, with two exceptions.

We were surprised to see it on the front page. Our impression from the reporters working on the story was that there was no inclination to hype it, and the text itself was on the whole well balanced, pointing out that there was no independent confirmation for the charges. But placement on the front page said to any sophisticated reader that the *New York Times* thought this was something big.

The other surprise was the misleading description of the sources of the story. The *Times* said it had come from "sources close to the investigation." This was both true and extremely deceptive. Although I did not know all the details then, I later learned from people at the *Times* that their source was none other than Roy Cohn, defense counsel for Steve Rubell.

The *Times* knew that its original source was by no means a disinterested party. But that information was not passed on to its readers.

According to reporters at the *Times*, Cohn originally took the story to his friend William Safire. Safire dashed off a memo. When things did not move quickly enough to suit him, Cohn called *Times* Executive Editor Abe Rosenthal, who made no secret of his dislike for Jimmy Carter and his administration.

With that knowledge, neither the disingenuous description of sourcing nor the front-page play are a mystery. Had I known at the time of the roles and relationships of Rosenthal, Safire, and Cohn, I would have been even more worried and less inclined to cooperate with the *Times*.

From that point on, little that was positive or encouraging happened for nine months, until Hamilton was finally cleared by a special prosecutor and a federal grand jury.

There were a few light moments. Shortly after the story broke, we began to hear that Studio 54's regular jet-set clientele was in a state of wrist-flapping hysteria. We were not surprised a few days later to see Rona Barrett reporting from Hollywood on *Good Morning America* that she had just spoken with Roy Cohn, and he had assured her that no names of celebrities who had used drugs at Studio 54 would be given to the Justice Department.

By mid-September the news coverage had begun to taper off. The *Times* had reported Johnny C., the drug pusher that Rogovin and Cohn claimed as an eyewitness to the incident, had denied to the FBI that he had ever been present that night, much less given any cocaine to Jordan. A change of their story by the accusers, removing me from the scene, had let me get back to my regular responsibilities as spokesman on the issue.

We also discovered that Rubell had attempted to pass on a fabricated story to John Fairchild of Fairchild Publications more than a year earlier. Rubell told Fairchild on August 8, 1978, that "Jordan and Powell" had visited Studio 54 on the previous evening and asked "if they could get some stuff and see some girls." Fairchild checked and found that Hamilton and I had been in Washington on August 7 and 8. When Fairchild confronted Rubell with this fact, he backed down, saying that perhaps it had been two people who looked like Jordan and Powell.

We gave this information to the *Times*. After a delay of three days it appeared in print, along with a list of other inconsistencies and contradictions in the statements from Hamilton's accusers. Unfortunately, that story ran on page 18. The contrast with the placement of the original accusations on page 1 exacerbated our suspicions and paranoia.

Still, the coverage seemed to be swinging our way. Then on September 11, as the FBI was about to dispose of the Studio 54 case, Mitchell Rogovin brought a new set of allegations to the Justice Department, thus precipitating a new investigation. The charges were based upon statements from a troubled woman in Los Angeles, who recanted as soon as her accusations became public, and statements from Leo Wyler and Harold Willens, two outspoken political enemies of the President, who were unable to provide any specific information about anything.

The substance of the California charges evaporated quickly, but they are interesting for two reasons.

They provided a glimpse of the conduct of Mitchell Rogovin. Shortly after he brought the allegations to the Justice Department, he leaked them to the press. Then he denied having brought them to Justice in the first place. Officials at Justice were so incensed that they told reporters Rogovin had lied to them. Unfortunately, but not surprisingly, reporters never wrote a word about the duplicity of their source. In its front-page story, the *New York Times* claimed not to know who had brought the allegations to Justice. As in the case of the initial story from Cohn, the *Times* coverage implied that the source was neutral and unbiased when exactly the reverse was true.

As I was to discover later, this was not the only or the most startling example of questionable behavior by Rogovin. Throughout the entire process, he claimed that he had brought the Studio 54 allegations to Justice in a traditional attempt to plea-bargain— "Go easy on our clients and they will give you incriminating information on someone more important."

What he actually tried to do was subtly but significantly different—so different that former Attorney General Civiletti characterizes it as "blackmail." He and U.S. Attorney Fiske say that Rogovin came to them not with an offer to cooperate, but with a threat. The message was in effect, "We have damaging information about a high government official; we'll tell no one but you if you'll give our clients a break. If not, we'll go public, and there will be severe political and national security implications."

Mr. Rogovin is not the first lawyer to attempt to blackmail his government in an effort to obtain leniency for a criminal. He may be the first former official of the IRS and the CIA to indulge in such tactics. He is now engaged in the private practice of law in Washington. His annual income is somewhat in excess of the legal bills Hamilton Jordan is still trying to pay.

The second noteworthy aspect of the California charges is the press coverage they spawned in their brief existence. It was the most sensational and irresponsible coverage of the entire nine months, and the worst example appeared on none other than the *CBS Evening News*, with Walter Cronkite.

About four o'clock on the afternoon of September 20, I took a call from Bob Pierpoint of CBS. He seemed a bit uncomfortable, which was unusual for the most experienced network correspondent at the White House. It did not take long to find out why. He said that CBS would be running interviews that night containing damaging accusations about Hamilton's behavior at a party in Los Angeles, including charges that he used drugs. He wanted an interview with Hamilton to respond to the charges.

I asked for a transcript of the interview. None was available. I asked for the specifics of the charges: where, when, who had made them. Bob did not know, and he was unable to hide his discomfort at being placed in such an awkward position. After a call back to CBS, he was able to tell me enough to make it clear that the allegations were similar, if not identical, to those that Rogovin had brought to the Justice Department a week earlier and that had been running for the past several days in the *Washington Post*, the *Los Angeles Times*, the *New York Times*, and particularly the *Los Angeles Herald-Examiner*.

We had decided early in the fight not to place Hamilton in the position of responding publicly, particularly on camera, to every charge that was made. There were several reasons for this decision. The first was legal. Since the matter could, and eventually did, end up before a grand jury, Ham's lawyers did not want him making a series of public comments.

In addition, we had learned through bitter experience that the perpetrators of this scheme could and would use information we provided in Hamilton's defense to concoct new stories. When we attacked the credibility of the original Studio 54 allegations by pointing out factual errors—I had never been to Studio 54, and neither Hamilton nor I were in New York in April of 1978 when, Rogovin originally said, the events took place—Cohn and Rogovin produced a new "witness" who told a different story to accommodate the accurate information we had provided. We were helping them perfect their charge, and they seemed to be suffering little or no loss in their ability to obtain attention from the press due to the errors and inconsistencies we pointed out.

We had also been worried about establishing a pattern of responding to every charge, which could come back to haunt us if we were faced with a collection of vague innuendos that could not be refuted quickly because of their generalized nature. We now faced a classic example of that situation.

I told Pierpoint that I doubted we would want to put Hamilton in front of a camera to respond to the allegations, but could not say for sure without more information. After several conversations in which Pierpoint acted as a messenger between me and Sandy Socolow, who was at that time the executive producer of the *CBS Evening News*, I began to get enough of a feel for the story to be worried and even more unsure about how we could respond. However, my conviction that we should not throw Hamilton into the midst of all this became stronger.

Finally, Pierpoint suggested that I come back to the CBS booth and talk directly with Socolow by phone. After listening to him describe their story, I exploded. All it boiled down to was two avowed political opponents of the President claiming that some people with Hamilton had behaved in a boisterous manner and that they had said some things that sounded as though they were talking about drugs. Socolow acknowledged that no one had claimed to have seen Hamilton or anyone else use drugs.

I knew from having dealt with a similar story in the *Los Angeles Herald-Examiner* a few days earlier that a number of people who had attended the party in question would state that they had witnessed nothing improper in Hamilton's behavior, much less anything that implied the use of drugs. I begged Socolow not to run the story until he had interviewed them.

He insisted that the CBS story did contain new and important material, and it would run that night to protect their exclusive. He would make the same argument three years later. In his view, CBS was being more than fair by offering Hamilton a chance to come on camera and respond to the innuendos.

By that time it was almost 6 P.M. I gave up on trying to get them to delay the story and raced back to the press office, where Rex Granum had been collecting the material we had used to deny the *Herald-Examiner* story. Pierpoint, who had been listening to my conversation with Socolow, was now visibly embarrassed and almost apologetic. If we could get him the information, he said, he would try to get as much of our response on the air as he could.

The story of the Los Angeles party was the lead item of the

CBS news broadcast that evening. It ran for more than six minutes, over one fourth of their entire broadcast, making it one of their biggest stories of the year.

I had walked around to Hamilton's office in the opposite corner of the West Wing to watch the news with him. His two lawyers happened to be there also. We were all shaken by what we saw. Hamilton and Steve Pollak typically had little to say. Henry Ruth and I paced the floor, occasionally cursing at the television set and speculating on the probable ancestry of various employees of CBS News.

Looking back on it, all four of us remember that evening as the most depressing point of the entire episode. Never at any other time during four years in the White House did I feel so useless and helpless. The story should never have been aired. It was as damaging as it was unfair. But I had been able to do absolutely nothing about it. For the first time, I thought that Hamilton might be forced to resign by negative press coverage before his innocence could be established.

There was almost nothing positive about the story. Pierpoint did point out in his closing segment that there were "at least three witnesses who were at the party who directly contradict descriptions of the party as licentious and say they saw no use of drugs." We also learned for the first time what CBS thought was so new and important about their story, what they were afraid their competitors would discover if they waited one day to check the story further: it was Willens's claim that he had brought his concerns to the attention of someone who worked in the White House.

The truth was that he had spoken with presidential adviser Dr. Peter Bourne, but he had made no mention of drugs and no specific references to any misbehavior on Hamilton's part. He had merely expressed his distaste for what he considered to be "licentious behavior" on the part of a group of people who had come to his party. Hamilton had been a member of that group. Bourne says the subject was mentioned only briefly, and Willens did not seem to attach particular importance to it. It was one of about two dozen things they talked about during the course of the conversation, according to Bourne.

As for the claim that this was news, the *Herald-Examiner* had reported Willens's contact with the White House on September

17, three days earlier, and CBS knew it. Mike Wallace, who conducted the interview with Willens and Wyler, says he specifically remembers reading that story. In fact, Wallace says it prompted him to arrange to have lunch with the reporter who wrote it and to seek the interviews with Wyler and Willens.

As for his refusal to hold the story for a day so others at the party could be interviewed, Socolow says, "Generally, the only times I have gotten into trouble have been when I held off. . . . When you have a story, you go with it; otherwise, you are in deep trouble. This one was ready, except for the rebuttal testimony. Frankly, I wasn't sure I would ever get it."

Socolow still has no regrets about the way the story was handled. Others at CBS were not, and are not, so sanguine. They are reluctant to speak for the record now, as they were then. But two of them called the day after the story ran to express sympathy and to apologize.

One, who was out of town and did not see the story until several days later, says he remembers thinking, "How could something like this have gotten on the air?" Another now says, "Everyone knew we had screwed up bad even before the show was over."

After his retirement, Walter Cronkite told friends that he considered the handling of this story "one of the most regrettable episodes" and "worst mistakes" of his entire career. Looking back on it, Cronkite has said to me that he cannot think of any story he misjudged more.

In Cronkite's defense, others at CBS point out that he was at a luncheon with CBS corporate executives that day until midafternoon. By the time he returned, Socolow was "set in concrete" on the decision to use and lead with the story. Cronkite, who had the authority to overrule Socolow, raised some questions, but let the decision stand.

Listening to Cronkite's reflections three years later, I began to develop a sick feeling in the pit of my stomach. What if I had talked to him instead of Socolow; might that have made a difference?

"I don't know," he said. "Maybe. In any case, you should have tried."

He was right; I should have.

"NEVER APOLOGIZE, NEVER EXPLAIN!"

I witnessed no more glaring example of the unwillingness of the fourth estate to find anyone innocent than an encounter with ABC News in the late summer of 1979. In this case, the problem was that ABC had already announced that the party was guilty. And the falsely accused, innocent party was the government of the United States.

The words of advice that form the title of this chapter were supposedly first spoken by a politician when asked how to deal with accusations of wrongdoing from either the media or political opponents. His name has, so far as I can tell, been lost to history. There may be a lesson in that.

For public officials accused of a mistake or worse, refusing to apologize or explain is usually a recipe for disaster, particularly if the accusation is false. But there is one powerful institution in our society that still lives by that rather arrogant and amoral precept, lives by it and prospers. It also happens to be the institution that does most of the accusing of everybody and everything else: the fourth estate.

What follows is an account of one of the most blatant examples of the "never apologize" mode of behavior. It is also an example of some of the weaknesses in journalism that help to create those errors that seldom are retracted or even acknowledged.

The latter part of August in 1979 was a hectic and not very happy time for the Carter administration. The press was at the height of its "The people want Teddy" frenzy. In addition, we were dealing with the accusations of cocaine use against Hamilton

Jordan, a confrontation with the Soviet Union over an on-again-off-again defection by a ballerina, a grand jury investigation of charges instigated by Jack Anderson that Jordan and Charles Kirbo were involved in underhanded dealings with Robert Vesco, and a controversy over a meeting between UN Ambassador Andrew Young and an official of the Palestine Liberation Organization. (Such meetings were prohibited by a commitment to the Israeli government made by Henry Kissinger during the Sinai withdrawal negotiations. The commitment has been restated by all subsequent Presidents.)

This particular incident brought about Young's resignation from the administration. It was a tragic and painful event for all concerned.

The Young controversy was also the basis for a story about U.S. intelligence-gathering activities that reflected extreme discredit on high government officials from the President on down. It alleged that the U.S. government was in violation of its own laws. Worse, it was completely false from start to finish.

That story is the subject of what follows. Not only was it wrong, but the news organization that broadcast it had been told it was wrong before it was aired. To make matters worse, many at ABC became convinced that it was wrong shortly thereafter, but the network has never, to this day, been willing to retract the charges, much less explain or apologize.

On August 29, 1979, ABC's *World News Tonight* led with a report that "ABC News has learned" that "U.S. intelligence agencies bugged the residence of UN Ambassador Andrew Young." It was this bug, ABC explained, that had tipped the State Department to Young's plans to meet with the PLO official.

Whether that meeting was also bugged, said ABC ominously, "is not clear." But there was no doubt, said the report, that an earlier meeting between Young and the Kuwaiti ambassador, where the PLO meeting was arranged, had been bugged by American intelligence services.

Before that report went on the air, ABC had flat denials from Attorney General Civiletti and FBI Director Webster, the only two officials who could authorize bugging. ABC ran with the story anyway, claiming that it "had been confirmed" by several other officials, which was untrue. Not until their second feed (the networks commonly feed to their affiliates two evening news programs, one at six-thirty and another, updated version at seven) was there any mention of the denials from Civiletti and Webster.

And even then ABC altered the statement that had been carefully read to them. When it was broadcast, it became a denial that the Attorney General and the FBI director had *"any knowledge"* of the bugging, when in fact the statement had actually said, without any equivocation, that *there had been no bugging*, period.

Shortly after the broadcast aired, I issued a denial on behalf of the President, and warned the other two networks, the wires, and major newspapers to stay away from ABC's story, which they did.

The next morning the President, who had ordered a survey of all intelligence agencies out of an abundance of caution, stared straight into the ABC cameras and stated flatly, and with some heat, that the story was "wrong and irresponsible" and that ABC knew it was wrong when they put it on the air.

All other news organizations were shunning the story like the plague. But ABC's people were determined not to let it go. It was repeated several times on their morning news program, broadcast throughout the day over their radio network, and repeated again on the evening news.

This time a host of denials, including the President's, were used. However, ABC attempted to vindicate its position by claiming that the story had been "confirmed by a high-ranking government spokesman" and that the first denials had come after the story was broadcast. Both those contentions were false.

ABC closed its second evening news story on the bogus bugging by stating enigmatically that its investigation was continuing. That investigation may be the longest in journalistic history. In the more than four years since that night, not one word has ever been mentioned on ABC News about the alleged bugging of Andy Young.

What were ABC's viewers and listeners supposed to think? They had been told repeatedly over a twenty-four-hour period that the U.S. government had bugged the residence of its ambassador to the United Nations. Not "may have" or "is alleged to have," which would have been bad enough, but "did." Flat, absolute, without question.

These viewers and listeners then heard denials from an impressive array of top officials, but no indication that ABC had any doubt about the accuracy of its allegations. Indeed, the clear implication of the final story was that the President and the others might well be lying.

Then they were told that an investigation was under way, presumably to resolve the matter. Then nothing.

How this came about says a great deal about news gathering, and not just television news gathering. But more than that, it is a demonstration of the casual arrogance of unfettered power, answerable to no one but the Almighty and congenitally incapable of admitting a mistake.

It all began, as do many Washington scoops, not with surreptitious phone calls or clandestine meetings in basement garages, but with an overheard and half-understood conversation at a cocktail party.

During the weekend before the story aired, Dan Brewster, a young and relatively inexperienced writer for ABC News, was at a cocktail party where he heard, or thought he heard, that the U.S. government had learned of Andy Young's meeting with the PLO representative through "intelligence sources."

That happened to be good information, and not a bad story in itself. But Brewster's inexperience, and perhaps an inclination to make a good story better, led him to surmise that this must mean that the Carter administration had sicced the FBI on its own ambassador, who also happened to be black, and a former civil rights worker, and a close associate of Martin Luther King, Jr., and wow!

Brewster had what might turn out to be a ticket to instant fame and glory. He persuaded his bureau chief to allow him to work on the story, but he was warned that he would need several sources before ABC would even think about airing such a report. Unfortunately, that warning turned out to be hollow.

On Monday, Brewster went to Hodding Carter, spokesman for the State Department (the original story about Young's ill-advised meeting had come from State, and Brewster's overheard conversation had been between State Department officials). Brewster said he had learned that Ambassador Young's apartment had been bugged.

Carter was faced with a difficult dilemma. He knew that there had been intelligence reports indicating that Young had met with the Kuwaiti ambassador and discussed with him plans to meet privately with the PLO representative. He also knew that this report had not been derived from the bugging of the Andy Young apartment or from any other type of spying on Young by any U.S. intelligence agency.

He could confirm the existence of intelligence reports, but he could not disclose where they had come from.

The same dilemma confronted Justice Department spokesman Terry Adamson when he was contacted by Brewster the next day. What both spokesmen did was to confirm in effect the existence of intelligence reports, but refuse to comment on how they had been obtained.

This refusal to discuss "sources and methods" was completely legitimate. Its purpose was to protect a valuable source of intelligence that might well have been jeopardized by revelation. Furthermore, these sources and methods involved no degree of wrongdoing by the United States government, under even the strictest interpretation of legal and ethical standards.

Had Brewster been experienced in the intelligence field, he would *not* have assumed that what he had received was a tacit admission that the U.S. government had bugged Andrew Young's apartment. But that is just what he did. Nor would he have assumed, as he clearly did throughout, that bugging Young was the only way, or even the most likely way, that U.S. intelligence agencies could have learned of Young's conversation with the Kuwaiti ambassador.

Following his conversations with Adamson, Brewster informed his superiors at ABC that the required confirmations were now in hand. They had come from no less than the spokesmen for the Secretary of State and the Attorney General.

At which point ABC demonstrated the inverted priorities of the news business. Brewster's story was turned over to Tim O'Brien, the regular Justice Department correspondent, to report on the evening news.

The most crucial part of the job, the reporting and checking of the story, had been quite all right for an inexperienced, young reporter with no background in the area in which he was dealing.

Now that inexperienced reporting had produced what appeared to be confirmation, a more senior, better-known personality had to be called in to appear on camera. Tell me it ain't show biz.

O'Brien was given the story shortly after five o'clock in the afternoon. He had almost no time to do any checking for himself. He did, however, call Terry Adamson, whom he had been interviewing at some length on an entirely different matter just a few minutes earlier. But then O'Brien had been working on a report on the Special Prosecutor's Act. He had no idea that the bugging story was in the works, because no one at ABC had bothered to tell him.

When O'Brien called, Adamson says, he was clearly seeking neither explanation nor confirmation, but a comment. Adamson, who had not suspected that ABC would actually air such a story during his conversations with Brewster, now realized that matters were getting out of hand.

He immediately placed a call to FBI Director Webster. They agreed that a strong and unequivocal statement of denial was needed urgently.

While it was being drafted, a friend at ABC called to tell him that his "no comments" were being taken as a confirmation by ABC and that the story was to lead the evening news. Adamson asked to speak to Brewster and told him that a strong denial was coming momentarily and he had better not make any accusations about the FBI or the Justice Department bugging Young.

Brewster suggested that the bugging may have been done by "other American intelligence agencies," an unlikely idea to anyone familiar with American intelligence procedures or the laws that govern them. Adamson said he obviously could not speak for the whole government, which was true, but an unequivocal denial from Justice was coming shortly. He had earlier explained to Brewster that the FBI was the only U.S. intelligence agency that was empowered to conduct such surveillance and then only under certain explicit rules and regulations.

He also pointed out that his earlier statements could hardly be confirmation of an alleged act of illegal surveillance that neither he nor the Attorney General knew anything about. (This last point—that the response from Justice might, at most, be interpreted as less than a complete denial but certainly not as any sort of confirmation—was apparently lost on Brewster and everyone else at ABC until the next day, when Adamson pointed out the logical fallacy in their reasoning.)

The formal denial was read directly to Brewster by FBI spokesman Homer Boynton at 5:35. It said: "Any implication that United States Ambassador Andrew Young was the subject of FBI surveillance or investigation is untrue."

O'Brien by that time had written his script and was on his way over to see Adamson at the Justice Department. Brewster said later that he took the denial to anchorman Frank Reynolds. Reynolds claimed that he never saw it.

When O'Brien showed Adamson what he planned to say, Adamson was appalled. "You don't even have the right Attorney General!" he exclaimed. Indeed, in his haste to put the story together at the last minute, O'Brien had used the name of the present Attorney General, Ben Civiletti, instead of that of Griffin Bell, who had held the office when the bugging allegedly took place.

While Adamson and O'Brien were talking, Civiletti walked into Adamson's office unannounced. He proceeded, in Adamson's words, to "deny the story in all particulars." Adamson remembers saying repeatedly, "It [the story] is absolutely wrong."

But O'Brien concluded that the Attorney General, and presumably Adamson too, was not telling the truth. He would later say to Adamson, "Our story is right. Ben Civiletti knows it is right. [He] is lying, and I can prove it."

As a result, the only change made in the story was to add a statement to the effect that high Justice officials, including the Attorney General, denied any knowledge of the bugging of Andrew Young's apartment.

This was particularly disingenuous, implying as it did that the bugging had in fact taken place, and changing Civiletti's denial "in all particulars" to a weak disclaimer of any knowledge of the act.

To be as charitable as possible to ABC, one can understand, if not excuse, what happened on that first afternoon and evening. The mistakes made were obvious and serious:

- An inexperienced reporter was assigned to deal with an important and explosive story that touched upon extremely complicated and sensitive matters.

- The refusal of government spokesmen to comment on intelligence sources and methods was taken as confirmation of what the reporter wanted to believe.

- Brewster failed to tell Reynolds, or anyone else, exactly what it was Hodding Carter and Terry Adamson had said that he considered to be a confirmation. And neither Reynolds nor anyone else at ABC bothered to ask.

- A somewhat more experienced reporter, albeit one whose reputation included a penchant for sensationalism, was not assigned until the last minute.

- There may have been a breakdown in communications between Brewster and Reynolds on the FBI denial.

- Faced with a choice between totally retracting a story that had already gone out on their early feed and assuming that the Attorney General was a liar, O'Brien and his colleagues chose the latter.

To that list may be added two other sins:

- ABC failed to involve John Scali, their one reporter with impeccable intelligence-community connections. If there was a suspicion that the surveillance had been conducted by some agency other than the FBI, he was by far the best person to run it down.

- ABC also failed to bring their White House correspondents into the story. Again, if someone thought that the Justice Department denials were limited to activities of that department and the FBI, the place to go for a comment that would deal with all activities and agencies was the White House.

Still, both Terry Adamson and Hodding Carter say that in retrospect they wish they had handled the matter differently. Both say that had they ever dreamed that ABC would air a story based only on the reporting of a young reporter neither had ever seen before, they would have, in Adamson's words, "screamed at Brewster a bunch of unprintables denying all semblance of his story."

Whatever judgment one makes about the events leading up to the first story—and it is possible, if one wishes to be extremely generous, to see how ABC might have thought there was something there—the behavior of ABC after it was aired is by no stretch of the imagination understandable, except in the context of arrogant and irresponsible refusal to acknowledge error.

As has been noted, I issued a comprehensive denial on the President's behalf late on the evening of August 29. The President himself publicly repudiated the story on the morning of the thirtieth. At about the same time Frank Reynolds, O'Brien, and ABC bureau chief George Watson met with Adamson at the Justice Department, presumably as part of their "continuing investigation."

At that meeting, Adamson was surprised to learn that they had not one bit of evidence to support their story except for the conclusion by Brewster that it had been confirmed by Adamson and Carter.

Reynolds insisted that the refusal to comment could legitimately be taken as a confirmation. Maybe and maybe not, but neither he nor Watson was able to explain away the later, unequivocal denials from the FBI and Civiletti.

Clearly upset, they warned Adamson that if they were forced to retract they would identify him and Hodding Carter as the officials who had confirmed the story. He responded heatedly that he was not afraid of a fight and that if such a story was aired, he would pursue legal remedies, including a suit for libel and a request for equal time. In addition, he promised to make public the entire series of exchanges between him and ABC, declaring that the result would certainly be to make ABC out as "the most ridiculous and irresponsible [news] organization of all time." An overstatement, perhaps, but not by much.

Whatever the reason, ABC did not attack Adamson and Carter by name that night. However, they repeated the charges and insisted that they had been "confirmed . . . by a high-ranking government spokesman." No mention was made of the fact that the confirmation was actually a "no comment," nor that the spokesman had clearly not intended his failure to comment to be taken as a confirmation, nor that this questionable confirmation was the only substantiation for the story.

Perhaps the most devious statement of all was the claim that an investigation was continuing. There was no further investigation. Scali was never called in to check his sources, perhaps because they had already called him to deny the story and protest vigorously and Scali had relayed their views along with his own condemnation of the report to his superiors.

To this day, no one at ABC can provide one shred of evidence that was collected from anyone after the announcement of a continuing investigation was aired.

Indeed, there was apparently no real inclination to check up on their story with a view toward correcting it if it could not be substantiated. Rather the opposite. Frank Reynolds was reported to have said, in explanation of why the story was never retracted, "I've never been persuaded that the report we gave was in error, therefore there is no need to correct the record."

That, my friends, is one of the more remarkable statements ever uttered by a responsible journalist. The burden of proof, once the story is aired, shifts to the injured party. It is, according to ABC, the responsibility of the government to prove that an event did not occur. This is both a logical impossibility and a complete inversion of the accepted standards of journalism.

Perhaps such an attitude would have been defensible if ABC had had some hard evidence, even an anonymous statement from an official in a position to know, to the effect that the bugging had taken place. But they did not. All they had was an assumption that "no comment" meant "yes."

Not everyone at ABC was happy with such behavior. Executives and reporters have told me since then that the clear consensus among those involved was that the story had been in error. When asked why the public was never informed of this conclusion, they can only shrug and say, as one did to me, "That's just the way this business works. You ought to know that by now."

Postscript: How did we learn of the planned meeting? That information is still classified and appropriately so. The sources and methods are still in use and would be damaged, if not destroyed, by public disclosure. Suffice it to say that the President, the Attorney General, the director of central intelligence, and this writer all state again that no bugging of Andrew Young's apartment nor any other illegal activity by any agency of the American government was involved.

Back to you, ABC.

A NEAR
MISS _____

A point to remember is that while the print and broadcast media often get carried away with stories of personal scandal, and run stories without sufficient corroboration, they do not run everything they are told. This is what happened with a story that alleged White House staff members were involved with drugs and homosexuality. It never appeared. And it is an example of how terribly damaging rumors can be passed on and given credence by individuals, including law enforcement officials, who have acted without apparent malice.

On August 17, 1979, Alan Baron, a well-known Washington political activist and publisher of a newsletter, was arrested and charged with possession of cocaine with intent to distribute. The news of his arrest was prominently displayed in both the *Washington Star* and the *Washington Post*.

Baron had worked for a number of liberal Democrats, including George McGovern and Morris Udall during their presidential campaigns. He had been made executive director of the Democratic party after McGovern won the Democratic nomination in 1972, but was replaced in '73 when Robert Strauss became the party chairman. Baron's newsletter, which capitalized on his extensive contacts, was considered to be among the more insightful in Washington.

Baron's arrest came at the end of an investigation that began in July of 1979 when an informant tipped a narcotics squad detective that Leonard Frank Ball, a Washington lawyer, was selling cocaine. A buy was arranged and Ball was arrested. Two weeks later, Ball agreed to identify his supplier in return for having the charges against him dismissed. The name he gave to the police was Kevin Goldstein, Alan Baron's roommate. A raid on Goldstein's apartment resulted in the arrest of both Baron and Goldstein. (Police told reporters that Baron had a vial containing half a gram of cocaine in his pants pocket when he was arrested.)

Shortly after his arrest, Baron told police that he had helped to obtain cocaine for Hamilton Jordan and Jody Powell, and that he knew them to be frequent users of the drug.

On August 26, the day after the Studio 54 story broke in the *New York Times*, a D.C. narcotics detective passed along the Baron allegations to *Post* reporters. The detective also said that one of the items confiscated in the raid on the Baron-Goldstein apartment was a notebook containing names, addresses, and phone numbers of senators, congressmen, journalists, and White House officials, including Powell and Jordan. He suggested that the names might be connected to drug sales and/or to a male prostitution ring that operated out of the same building. The notebook, according to the detective, was locked in an evidence locker. He could not get his hands on it without arousing suspicion. However, he promised to make a copy for the reporters later. In the meantime, Baron told the *Post* the same story he had told police—that he had helped Jordan and Powell obtain cocaine.

The charges touched off a flurry of investigative activity, the intensity of which was heightened by the appearance of the Studio 54 charges in the *New York Times*. Dozens of phone calls were placed to White House staffers and to their friends, inside and outside of government, to try to find someone who had seen Hamilton or me use cocaine. At one point, two reporters toured the city's gay bars, seeking information that would confirm the allegations and trying to track down the original informant.

The informant was eventually located by *Post* reporters at his parents' home in Brunswick, Maryland. His name was John Conners, and he was familiar to the reporters because he had accused a congressman of homosexual rape several months earlier. (The congressman admitted to reporters that he had picked Conners up in a gay bar and had sex with him, but denied that rape was involved. No charges were ever brought.) However, Conners had no information about drug use by Hamilton or me or others on the White House staff.

The *Post* arranged interviews with the U.S. Attorney Charles Roistacher and with sources in his office. The Justice Department was called to see if they had heard of the charges against Hamilton and me.

Martin Schram, recently hired by the *Post* to cover the White House, was called into the story, as was Art Harris, a reporter who had once worked in Georgia and was thought by people at the *Post* to know a great deal more about "the Georgians" than he did.

At the White House, meanwhile, we were immersed in the Studio 54 allegations, plus the Soviet-brigade-in-Cuba flap, civil war and Israeli intervention in Lebanon, the publicity buildup for Ted Kennedy's announcement that he would run for the presidency, and energy legislation in the Congress. We were almost completely unaware of what the *Post* was up to. I assumed that the calls to White House staffers resulted from a spin-off to the Studio 54 stories. I accused the *Post* of embarking on a fishing expedition. I suggested that if they were interested in developing stories on drug use in Washington by calling people at random to ask if they had ever used drugs, they might start in their own newsroom.

Then during the first week in September, I heard that there might be some connection to the Baron case. I had paid little attention to it at the time, and could hardly remember it three weeks later. The rumors were vague and I dismissed them from my mind.

Had I known what the *Post* had and what they were trying to prove, I suspect I would have seriously considered suggesting to Hamilton that he take a leave of absence. I would have assumed that sooner or later the charges would be published and that Hamilton could not survive the increased pressure they would generate.

Fortunately, almost miraculously, it never came to that. By September 22, the *Post* had completed the circle. No one could be found who had seen anyone at the White House use cocaine.

The narcotics detective still claimed that at least one informant (Ball) said he had firsthand knowledge, but Ball himself denied knowing anything about it. He said that he had never told the police that he did.

Baron now admitted that he had no firsthand knowledge, but claimed he knew of two people who had been witnesses. However, he refused to give the reporters their names or to speak on the record.

Goldstein, through his attorney, told the *Post* that he "didn't know anything about the allegations."

The U.S. attorney's office and the Department of Justice reported that they had received no allegations. By then, because of the extensive coverage of the Studio 54 matter, even the most casual reader of the newspapers would have known that a full-scale investigation would be launched the minute any such charges were brought to the attention of the Justice Department.

The infamous notebook turned out to be Baron's address book, which he used to gather information for his newsletter. The phone numbers listed for Jordan and Powell were those of the White House switchboard.

What should the *Post* do now? Bob Woodward, the assistant managing editor in charge of the *Post* investigation, suggested that a story be written describing what had happened, making it clear that the original reports could not be verified, and explaining how unsubstantiated rumors could find their way into the press if great care was not taken to check them thoroughly. He thought this would be a useful story, given the amount of coverage the Studio 54 charges were receiving.

Others at the *Post* were hesitant. On the day the question was being discussed, an item appeared in William Safire's column in the *New York Times* implying that the D.C. Police Department was failing to pursue evidence of drug use in the White House. How would the *Post* look if they published a story saying there was nothing there, only to have another paper discover later that there was? It is, after all, impossible to prove a negative.

Woodward did not push his idea. He now says he wishes he had. Perhaps it would have caused other news organizations to be more careful in their handling of the Studio 54 and related allegations.

Still, it is remarkable and commendable that the *Post* showed as much restraint as it did. On other occasions, papers, including the *Post*, have published with no more to go on than the *Post* had. The competitive pressure that contributed to eagerness with which the *Times* pursued the Studio 54 story, and to the prominence of their coverage, was at a height during the investigation of Alan Baron's charges. Studio 54 was a *Times* story; what a coup it would have been for the *Post* to top it with another cocaine charge, this time with undertones of homosexuality.

However, before we become too complacent, it is worth noting that most of the reporters who worked on the story agree that had Baron been willing to speak on the record, his allegations would have been published, despite the lack of evidence to corroborate them. Had that happened, it is unlikely that Hamilton could have survived. My job would also have been in jeopardy. The fact that the charges turned out to be false would have made little difference in their immediate effect.

Thinking back on it all, Bob Woodward told me: "We are pretty good at investigating and nailing someone who is guilty. When we set our minds to it, we can do that, but we never find anyone innocent. If we can't verify an accusation, we just go on to the next one. I'm not sure that is the way it should be."

IN
RETROSPECT

T he events of Watergate, Vietnam, and that whole tur-
bulent decade of souring relations between press and government have created a residue of cynicism that is a
serious and corrosive force.

Listen to Bob Woodward talking about Hamilton Jordan and
cocaine: "You have to remember that our experience for the past
ten or fifteen years has been that in the end the government official always ended up being guilty as charged. We just didn't run
across people whose defense held up under close scrutiny."

Or to a reporter from the *New York Times* who worked on the
Jordan story, explaining in strikingly similar words why he was
inclined to believe that Hamilton was guilty as charged: "In every
case that I can remember, the politician turned out to be lying.
No matter how reasonable his defense sounded or how sympathetic he seemed at the time, in the end we found out it was all a
bunch of lies."

The other bit of residue from times past is heightened competition for stories of scandal and wrongdoing in government. Few
at the *New York Times* dispute the contention that their determination not to be beaten by the *Post* again on a White House scandal
story played a role in the decision to publish quickly and to give
extra prominence to the charges against Jordan.

That pressure is not confined to the *Times*. The networks are
also sensitive to charges that they neglected the Watergate story
for months, as is the White House press corps in general. Other
news organizations, from the weekly newsmagazines to the wire

services to regional papers with little or no ability to cover national stories themselves, have become more likely to run and to play up such stories.

The problem is exacerbated by the blurring of the line between hard news and gossip. The phenomenon is exemplified by the emergence of "lifestyle" sections in many papers, including the *Post*, which combine interesting and usually inoffensive features with questionable "personality" stories. It is personified by individual writers such as Rudy Maxa of the *Post* and Diana Mc-Clellan, a.k.a. "The Ear," originally with the *Washington Star*, then the *Post*, and now the *Washington Times*.

Except for concern for the excessively permissive standards of libel law, such writing is usually subjected to less strict editorial scrutiny than hard news.

The style of the writing used for these sections is also less constrained by standards of journalistic propriety. The reporter has greater freedom to damn or accuse through innuendo. (In our first year in Washington, for example, my wife and I went to the Kennedy Center one night to see a play with a couple we had met at church. On the way home we stopped for a bite to eat. Two days later the evening was described in a gossip column as "Jody Powell out carousing late with a crowd of his drinking buddies.")

That sort of writing may have a place in this world, though I am not sure where it is; but there is certainly no place for it in a publication that purports to be serious and wishes to be respected. If the President's senior aide grossly insults an ambassador's wife, it belongs in the front section of the paper, not tacked on at the end of an essentially frivolous piece about how many parties various administration officials attend and what anonymous Washington socialites think about it.

If an important government official spits on a woman in a bar, that is news and deserves to be treated and played as such, not stuck in a gossip column that escapes the scrutiny of the experienced news editors of the paper.

The same can be said for a variety of "gossip" stories not mentioned in this book: a false and outrageous allegation in the "Style" section of the *Post* that Zbigniew Brzezinski "playfully" unzipped his fly in front of a female reporter and then sent her a picture to commemorate the incident; or an item that appeared in the "Ear" column charging that President Carter had bugged Blair House, the official residence for visiting foreign leaders, and had continued the eavesdropping while President-elect and Mrs. Reagan were staying there. (Both stories were retracted, the Brzezinski story immediately but the Blair House story only after an incredible period of defensiveness and resistance.)

These things ought to be written for the news sections of the paper. If the staffer who comes up with the tip is incapable of that higher-caliber journalism, then he or she should not be dealing with that sort of story. Turn it over to a legitimate reporter.

For the news side, the basic criterion is whether an item is news, whether it is relevant to anything important. To be relevant, by definition, it must be true. For gossip columns, where the essential question is whether the item is interesting or titillating, accuracy is of less consequence. The distinction is important, but it has become blurred. Serious journalists have allowed their territory to be invaded by traffickers in rumor and innuendo—and some have lowered their own standards to compete with the invaders.

There is a place in journalism for most of the softer, feature articles that appear in the lifestyle sections of many newspapers. But I question whether there is any place in any decent news publication for gossip. If a newspaper feels compelled to compete for the supermarket tabloid dollar, a separate enterprise would be more appropriate than trying to toss just a limited amount of trash into the same pages that seek respect for accurate and insightful coverage of important matters.

From their viewpoint, editors often argue that readers treat those items that appear in places other than the news sections of the paper less seriously. There is some truth in that contention. But the audience for these stories is not always limited to those who read them in their original form. Because the items are published in reputable, Pulitzer Prize–winning newspapers, they are often picked up by the wire services, and occasionally by the networks, and distributed to additional millions of people who are unaware that these stories should be taken with a very large grain of salt.

Most of those who work for the wire services and the networks will admit that they can do little independent checking as to the veracity of an item before it is put on the wire or on the air. There was certainly none in the case of either the amaretto and cream or the pyramids story. The wires and nets do make decisions on what is relevant. They do not pick up every intriguing bit of gossip that appears. That helps some, but it is not enough. There is a difference in relevance and newsworthiness, between something that is true and something that has yet to be proven true.

A special word should be said here about the television networks, because of their tremendous power if for no other reason. Although there are notable exceptions, the networks are not, for the most part, in the investigative reporting business. They are not set up for it and do not devote substantial resources to it on a continuing basis. When they want to, they can divert people and resources and do a commendable job.

The problem comes when they decide to jump into it on the spur of the moment, as was the case with the awful CBS story on Jordan that ended up embarrassing CBS personnel from Cronkite on down. By their own admission, neither Mike Wallace, who did the story, nor Sandy Socolow, the producer of the evening news, had been following the story closely. That infamous piece, which led the Cronkite show, was little more than a television adaptation of a series that had run in the *Los Angeles Herald-Examiner*, a struggling paper that was known occasionally to go for the sensational in an attempt to boost circulation.

Wallace's sources were essentially those who had been interviewed by the *Herald-Examiner*. Indeed, he has said that he got the names of the people he interviewed from the reporter who wrote the *Herald-Examiner* story. Wallace had no research and no file on the story because he had not been covering it. He did not talk to any of the CBS reporters at the White House or the Justice Department who had been following the story for weeks. Nor did he attempt to contact the White House for our version of what happened, which might have helped him to frame more pointed questions for those he interviewed, or at least to evaluate their responses.

Wallace had gone to California to work on an unrelated story for *60 Minutes*, one of the notable exceptions to television's general lack of thorough investigative journalism. But his reporting on the

Jordan story was a far cry from the time, effort, and research that usually go into a *60 Minutes* piece (which some at CBS say is why *60 Minutes* "didn't want anything to do with it").

The result was a "news" piece that led the Cronkite show, but had not one item of new information in it. When informed for the first time, three years later, that the one bit of news he thought the piece contained had also been previously reported, Socolow was not particularly disturbed. "It was," he said, "the first time they had said any of this on camera."

The prosecution rests.

There are some equally unflattering points to be made about the role of those in the White House, including this writer.

The most damning in my opinion is a sin of omission. Those of us who held senior positions on the President's staff had reasons to suspect that some, primarily younger members of the staff in lower-ranking positions occasionally used marijuana and were not terribly discreet about it. Until an incident in August of 1978, when Dr. Peter Bourne was forced to resign in the midst of a controversy over the writing of an improper prescription and allegations of drug use among some White House staffers, we never made a serious effort to put a stop to it. There were warnings and reminders at staff meetings, but the issue was not pursued vigorously. We rationalized that because the practice was widespread among others in Washington, including congressional staffers and journalists, the problem was not that serious. We were wrong.

By the time the Studio 54 charges surfaced, many reporters knew that some Carter staffers smoked marijuana because, in some cases, they had smoked together. That reputation for improper and indiscreet behavior gave impetus to the Jordan story and lessened the credibility of his denial.

Ironically, Hamilton was known within the White House as one who took a very hard line on drug use of any sort and probably did more than any other member of the senior staff to warn junior members to stay away from drugs. But none of us did enough. We paid a heavy price for it.

My handling of both the pyramids and the amaretto and cream stories was also a costly mistake.

In dealing with the pyramids story, I failed to do my homework. As a result, I was not sure exactly what had happened. Although I accepted Hamilton's denial, the press sensed the lack of certainty in my responses to their questions.

The absolute first rule of dealing with a crisis of any sort, particularly one that involves allegations of misconduct, is to know as precisely as possible what you are facing. It is seldom enough to simply state that such and such did not happen. Even the worst of stories are seldom constructed from whole cloth. It is extremely helpful to know which elements are true and which are distorted or altogether false. A denial is much more credible if reporters following up on the original charge can be provided with some type of logical explanation of what did happen.

When faced with the amaretto and cream story, I did the homework but used the information stupidly. The fact was that the story had appeared in a gossip column and not one that the White House press corps considered to be a fount of reliable information. I could have taken advantage of this, but did not. The story demanded a response and an effective one, but not one that unnecessarily attracted more attention to the charge.

A more effective approach would have been to poke fun at the story:

> This story is not credible on its face since it is common knowledge that no one has ever consumed amaretto and cream and light beer [beer was known to be Hamilton's usual drink] at the same sitting and survived.

Or:

> We have checked with Guinness and they have no record of anyone ever being able to spit over the head of one person and down the dress of another twice in succession without missing. Unfortunately, they refuse to list Mr. Jordan in their next edition because Mr. Maxa's story fails to meet their standards for corroboration. If Mr. Maxa has any hard evidence that this incident actually took place, we hope he will contact the *Guinness Book of World Records* and the White House.

Followed by a brief, but firm, denial:

> Mr. Jordan says that no such incident took place. He was in-

volved in a brief and unpleasant encounter with a young woman at Sarsfield's, which he did not provoke and which was entirely verbal. We have spoken with a number of witnesses to the incident, including a bartender who saw the entire episode, and they confirm Mr. Jordan's statement.

If some reporters were determined to pursue the matter further, as some undoubtedly would have been, the statements from the bartender and other witnesses could have been made available at their insistence, preferably in a condensed form, unless, as is likely, some had insisted on seeing the complete and unabridged transcript.

The above is not a new idea. It is essentially what Rex Granum, my deputy, suggested at the time. He was unable to convince me because I had let my desire to strike a blow at Maxa and others of his ilk get in the way of what should have been my primary consideration, how to protect Hamilton.

I was less ill used than Hamilton, primarily because my job required me to spend a great deal of my time with one of the more talkative and socially active groups in Washington, the press. Hamilton was disinclined to do the same thing, because, I think, he did not want to appear to be meddling in my area. Also, it was not his nature.

In that sense, part of what happened to Hamilton was my fault. I should have insisted that he establish contacts, at least with the reporters covering the White House. If I had given that problem the attention it deserved, and the relationship between White House and press was my responsibility, Hamilton might have been spared a great deal of what befell him.

Before leaving this subject, I must reiterate that a major portion of the injustice done in the Studio 54 case to Hamilton and to the President he served had nothing to do with shoddy journalism, inept press secretaries, partisan politics, or overzealous bureaucrats. The culprit was the law, the Ethics in Government Act of 1978. It was passed with the best of intentions, but portions of it have had the worst of effects.

As originally passed, it deprived a host of federal officials of the basic protections of our system of justice. As I said earlier, if an allegation of wrongdoing (except for a "petty" offense) was made against one of them, an investigation had to be launched—no matter how incredible the source or how technical or improbable the charge. If, within ninety days, the investigation did not prove the suspect innocent—that's right, not guilty but innocent—a special prosecutor had to be named.

There are some who would argue that if Hamilton Jordan had taken one snort of cocaine, the most he would have been guilty of was willful insensitivity. I do not agree. The violation of the law by a high government official is a serious matter. But I do agree that a full-scale FBI investigation and the prospect of a special prosecutor were excessive and a waste of time.

Consider that the alleged offense was one that is almost never prosecuted, and one that would have been virtually impossible to prove in a court of law. Law enforcement officials I have talked to at every level agree that no prosecutor or law enforcement agency in the country would dream of pursuing such a case under ordinary circumstances. The only possible results of such an exercise are the diversion of FBI agents from serious matters and damage to an official's ability to do his job, even if innocent.

In 1981 a number of senior officials from both the Carter and the Reagan administrations appeared before congressional committees to suggest amendments to make the law more reasonable. At first there seemed to be little enthusiasm for action. I suggested that if the members of Congress felt the law was fair, they should bring themselves under its jurisdiction. If the *New York Times* was so convinced that the law was a good thing, as it claimed editorially, perhaps its publisher and two or three other senior officials, who are unarguably more powerful in shaping the course of the nation than 95 percent of those covered by the act, would volunteer to come under its sway.

I even promised to come up with a well-drafted, anonymous letter containing charges against any Timesman who was ready to accept the challenge. I guaranteed that it would be impossible to prove within ninety days that the accusation was false or frivolous, and a special prosecutor would be appointed.

Of course, to make things completely fair, the *Times* would want to make sure the target of my false accusation paid his legal bills out of his own pocket. No company lawyers, please. The fact that the journalists covered would almost certainly have higher salaries than any of the government officials, except perhaps the President and Vice-President, would be an additional disparity. But I was willing to let that pass for the moment.

Fortunately, the Congress acted in late 1982 to remove some of the worst abuses in the act. The hair-trigger provision was made more realistic; the number of officials covered and the duration of the coverage have been reduced.

A provision was also included to provide compensation for legal fees to officials falsely accused. Unfortunately, even though most of the impetus for this reform and the others mentioned above came from the injustice done to Hamilton Jordan, the reimbursement provision was not made retroactive. It is now less likely that the law will victimize innocent officials in the future. But the one real victim has been left to struggle with his legal debts, ignored by the legislative body that helped set the stage for the injustice.

On the journalistic side, the *Washington Post* has called for the inclusion of Hamilton in the relief provided by the new legislation—just as it called for revision of the law in the midst of the attacks on Jordan. The *New York Times*, which used the quirk of the law as a basis for its hyped coverage of the charges against Jordan, has remained silent on the question of whether he is entitled to relief—just as it earlier declared opposition to any change in the law.

TEDDY
AND THE PRESS_____

No single episode of the entire four years produced more frustration for me, politically and in our relationships with the press, than the long fight for the Democratic nomination with Senator Edward M. Kennedy. The causes of that frustration relate to Kennedy himself, to some of the more unattractive weaknesses of the fourth estate, and, of course, to my own misjudgments.

If someone proposed a political novel featuring a character with Kennedy's record of nonaccomplishment in the Senate—not to mention the personal baggage that he has acquired—who was nevertheless a perennial and serious candidate for the highest office in the land, it would be dismissed as impossibly fantastic. Yet we found ourselves, well before the midterm point in the Carter administration, reading excited and adoring speculation in the press about whether or not the savior from Massachusetts might consent to offer himself in service to his party and the nation by running against an incumbent President of his own party.

In the fall of 1978, the political tide in the nation was clearly running to the right at an accelerated pace, as it had been since before Carter's election. But the dominant question to be noodled over by many political columnists was whether Jimmy Carter would have enough sense to move left to head off a challenge from Senator Kennedy.

The relationship between the President and the then junior senator from Massachusetts had never been particularly warm. An incident that revealed much about, and I suspect helped to shape, the personal attitudes on both sides occurred toward the end of the primary season in 1976.

The Carter campaign was within a hair of having the nomination locked up, but was losing momentum. The papers were full of anonymous quotes from various leading Democrats about the desirability of what was variously described as a "Stop Carter" or "Anybody But Carter" movement. The organizers eventually settled on the latter, presumably because they liked the ABC acronym.

On the night of May 25, 1976, we were headed for defeats in three of six primaries, including Oregon, the only one that was a real contest. In that state we were in danger of running third behind Frank Church and a hastily organized write-in effort on behalf of Governor Jerry Brown. When the people of Oregon are willing to go out of their way to vote for a Californian instead of your candidate, you know you have problems.

We had traveled back to New York that evening in an attempt, largely successful, to focus attention on all six states, including Tennessee, Kentucky, and Arkansas, where we were sure to pile up tremendous majorities, rather than just on our dismal prospects in three states in the West.

I had agreed to let David Nordan, political editor for the *Atlanta Journal* and a longtime friend and adversary from the political wars in Georgia, spend some time in the candidate's suite as the returns came in. The arrangement was that he would not quote anything he overheard without my approval.

My intentions were acceptable, if not altogether unselfish: to take care of the hometown paper by giving David a little something extra. However, it was a foolish idea. The most important rule in establishing ground rules for journalists is not to tempt them beyond what they can bear, a maxim that I learned early and forgot repeatedly. David had been reasonably reliable about observing ground rules. But I was now putting him in a situation where he might well come up with something that neither he nor any other reporter could stand not to report.

Sure enough, at the top of my list of things to brief the candidate about was a statement from Senator Kennedy accusing Jimmy Carter of being "intentionally . . . indefinite and imprecise" on the issues. The comment was obviously designed to help fuel the Anybody But Carter movement, which had adopted the "fuzzy on the issues" charge as its rallying cry. And it seemed to be timed to take advantage of what was not going to be one of our better primary nights.

My immediate reaction when I heard of the Kennedy statement, earlier that day, had been to wonder how in the hell he thought he was in any position to criticize anybody about being indefinite and imprecise. For reasons that I am still not sure I completely understand, Kennedy's statement was much more irritating to me than anything that had come from Hubert Humphrey or Henry Jackson or Jerry Brown, or any of the others who were associated with the effort to deny Carter the nomination. I had the feeling that Jimmy Carter shared my general attitude toward Kennedy, a suspicion that was not alleviated by his reaction to the senator's barb.

When I related what the senator had said, Carter replied evenly that he was thankful he didn't "have to kiss Teddy Kennedy's ass to win the nomination." And it was clear that he meant every word of it.

As David knew, we had originally planned the 1976 campaign around the assumption that we would be running against George Wallace and Kennedy. We saw a chance to seize the middle ground and score better than expected against Kennedy in New Hampshire and then against Wallace in Florida two weeks later. When Kennedy pulled out in late 1974, we were actually, though perhaps foolishly, disappointed.

It did not sit well with us later when analysts began attributing Carter's success to, among other things, the good fortune that Senator Kennedy had graciously decided not to run. We knew, as did many of them, that Kennedy had gotten out primarily because of the negative reaction among so many Democrats to his campaign and fundraising appearances on behalf of other candidates during the 1974 congressional election campaign.

His intrusion into the race under those circumstances was particularly resented. I had said at the time of his withdrawal that he now had an interest in a Republican victory in 1976 if he planned to seek the presidency at some later date. He could hardly challenge a sitting President of his own party in 1980, I figured naïvely; and the Vice-President would be the heir apparent in 1984.

Needless to say, the suspicion that Senator Kennedy was not interested in seeing a Democratic President in the White House unless his name was Teddy, and that he was willing to promote that interest when he felt he could get away with it, was not dispelled by anything I saw over the next five years.

There was that, plus the congenital disinclination of a south Georgia farmboy to kowtow to some Massachusetts pol who had inherited everything he had, from his political career to his bank account. David knew this, so of course he put it all on the front page of the *Atlanta Journal* the next day.

When Nordan's story began to move over the AP, I went bananas. I was not sure who deserved to be shot first—Nordan, Carter, or me. The month before we had wallowed in ethnic purity for a full week and were still scraping the remnants from beneath our toenails and behind our ears. Now I was sure we were in the same sort of mess again.

As it turned out, I was completely mistaken. Carter made it clear, as soon as I raised the subject with him the next day, that he had no intention of apologizing, but he would not tell me how he intended to handle it. I would just have to wait for the press conference, already scheduled for later that afternoon.

What he did was to pass it off with a smile and the comment that he was not sure he could remember that portion of his conversation that evening.

As it turned out, that was the end of it as a public issue, but it foreshadowed the tone of the Carter-Kennedy relationship for three years—and then it got worse.

If Jimmy Carter was not going to "kiss Teddy's ass" as a candidate, he was even less likely to do so as President. He did not. Three years later, when a congressman asked what he would do if Teddy ran against him, he replied in the same tone of voice that he intended to "whip his ass." And he did, albeit at tremendous political cost.

Early in the administration, pollster and political strategist Pat Caddell wrote an analysis of the political contests we were entering. Among other things, he predicted that we would catch more hell, and earlier, from the liberal wing of our own party than from the Republicans.

Despite what turned out to be an overzealous effort at appeasement—primarily through the presidential endorsement of a flood of liberal legislation that had been backlogged by eight years of Nixon and Ford vetoes—the overwhelming majority of the criticism directed at Carter during his first year in office came from the Democratic left. A survey of press coverage during that period revealed that fully 75 percent of the critical comments reported came from Democrats, mostly from the liberal wing of the party.

We learned early that there was little to be gained from a public fight with the senator. He had among the Washington press corps one of the most loyal and effective claques in existence. Based upon a nucleus of journalists who had aspired to be knights at his big brother's round table, it had been nurtured and expanded by careful attention to the stroking and flattery that seem to work as effectively on reporters as on other mortals.

In normal times, their responsibility was to avoid saying anything bad about Teddy personally—keeping rumors about women and drugs out of the press, for instance—and to snipe occasionally at those who were causing or might cause the senator problems.

One of our earlier experiences with this group involved the question of judicial appointments. The President had maintained a firm belief since before he was elected governor of Georgia that one of the most important legacies of any Chief Executive is the appointment of judges. Toward the end of making sure that his record in this area was the best that he could make it, he established a list of standards and procedures to guide him and his Attorney General in making selections. He was even willing, on occasion and with mixed success, to challenge the recommendations of sitting senators when he felt they did not meet the criteria he had established.

In theory, the idea was roundly applauded by the press, and even encouraged in practice, at least until Mr. Kennedy sought an exception to the rules and failed to get it.

One of the standards is age. The reasoning behind it is primarily economic. To appoint a federal judge who is approaching retirement when other equally qualified choices are available is a rip-off of the taxpayers. It amounts to an unearned sinecure. In return for only a few years of work, the appointee will be awarded a handsome pension for life.

The appointment of a judge who will almost certainly leave the bench within a few years is, more important, a waste of a judicial appointment. A President is, in effect, opting for a two- or three-year impact instead of twenty or thirty.

The American Bar Association has long refused even to consider the qualifications of any person age sixty-five or older. Carter and most previous Presidents had adopted the standard, and Senator Kennedy seemed to endorse it—at least for everyone but himself.

In early 1979, Senator Kennedy recommended the appointment of his good friend, and an eminently qualified lawyer, Archibald Cox to the First U.S. Circuit Court of Appeals. (Cox had been solicitor general during the administration of President John Kennedy.) Attorney General Griffin Bell was surprised, since he knew that Cox, at age sixty-eight, was well beyond the cutoff point. He first assumed that the problem could be easily corrected with a private chat.

Not so. The senator knew very well how old Mr. Cox was, and what the rule said, but he insisted that an exception be made.

When I first learned of the controversy, it did not concern me particularly. Surely, I thought, the senator would not try to make it a public issue when his position was so weak.

Wrong. When the Attorney General refused to make an exception and the President backed him up, pointing out that similar requests from other senators had been denied, the story was leaked to the press. The coverage that followed paid little attention to the question of standards or consistency. For the most part, the matter was portrayed as a simple, straightforward conflict between a vindictive little redneck and the charismatic chairman of the Senate Judiciary Committee, who was seeking unselfishly to place a distinguished American on the federal bench.

This incident also tarnished what had been a surprisingly good relationship between Judge Bell and Senator Kennedy. Although there was a wide philosophical gulf between them, the Attorney General had reason to try to bridge the gap. He had run John Kennedy's campaign in Georgia in 1960 and had been appointed to the bench by President Kennedy. Bell had also come to Washington with the realization that Senator Kennedy would soon become chairman of the Judiciary Committee, as indeed he did in 1979 after the retirement of Senator James Eastland.

He was determined to establish a good working relationship, and proceeded to do so. The parting of the ways came in April of 1979, when the two were at a judicial conference in Williamsburg. Kennedy, who was still insisting that Cox be appointed and threatening to veto through senatorial courtesy any other person named to fill the vacancy, called the Attorney General to one side to make another pitch for his recommendation. When Bell again stated that he simply could not recommend that the President make an exception, the senator exploded. Turning red in the face, he began to shout and wave his arms. His language, while not profane, was abusive and, as far as the Attorney General was concerned, insulting.

Despite frequent slurs on his motivations emanating from the senator's staff, Judge Bell never mentioned Senator Kennedy's extraordinary outburst to the press.

The senator and his supporters also continued to portray the matter as simply a mean-spirited action by a politically vindictive President, although they knew that the decision had been made by the Attorney General and supported by the President.

Ironically, one of the favors Senator Kennedy demanded and got before he was willing to support the Democratic ticket in 1980 was the appointment of Steve Breyer, one of his Senate aides, to this same judicial post. Breyer was one of the last Carter appointees confirmed by the Senate before the administration left office.

I had become convinced in December of 1978 that we were likely to face a challenge from Senator Kennedy. The place was the Democratic midterm conference in Memphis. We had known for some time that we were going to have trouble with the left wing of the party. The question was whether Kennedy would encourage or even lead the incipient rebellion. My expectation was that he would encourage it, but from a distance.

Wrong again. The senator arrived in Memphis with the clear intention of making sure that the news from this gathering of Democrats was dissatisfaction with the Carter administration. He had a fair amount of material to work with and he succeeded admirably. His public statements were largely devoid of any criticism of the Republicans. His attacks on Carter were indirect but unmistakable.

At one point he seized upon a recommendation to eliminate some duplications in the school lunch program. The Carter administration, he charged, was trying to take milk from the mouths of the schoolchildren of America.

Our attempts to explain the actual impact of the proposal, which stood little chance of clearing Congress anyway, were to no avail. Such an absurd bit of demagoguery from almost any other American politician would have been treated with open contempt by most journalists. But this was not any American politician, and his rhetoric was treated as serious and thoughtful analysis.

His principal theme at the convention was national health insurance. He insisted that the President endorse a comprehensive plan to be funded entirely from the federal treasury, warning that failure to do so could "split the Democratic party."

We tried to point out the tremendous cost of the senator's plan, that he had been unable for years to get it out of the heavily Democratic subcommittee he chaired, and that for him to accuse Carter of splitting the party was somewhat disingenuous—all to no avail.

Kennedy left before the principal vote of the conference, which was on two competing budget resolutions, one of which had been drafted for the express purpose of embarrassing the President. His partisans worked hard for the anti-administration resolution and to prevent any compromise that would avoid a confrontation.

We won the vote anyway, and also a CBS survey of presidential preference, by large margins. Nevertheless, the political analysis on the networks and in print was that Carter might have "controlled" the organization, but Kennedy had won the "cheers" and "hearts" of the delegates.

Beginning then and running through the first half of 1979, the line fed to the press by Senator Kennedy and his people was that he did not want to run, but might be forced into it by Carter's political weakness and/or his lack of ideological purity on the issues that were closest to the senator's heart.

Although I thought it was pure baloney, I had to give them credit for a skillful bit of design and salesmanship, because the normally cynical press swallowed it whole without gagging even once. Several reporters liked this analysis so much that they adopted it as their own without so much as a hint of its origins.

This placed us in an awkward position. If we tried to cuddle up to Kennedy on issues such as national health insurance, we would increase our vulnerability from the center and right, thus lending credence to Kennedy's "political weakness" argument. If we stuck to our guns, he would continue to accuse us of insensitivity to the poor, exacerbate our difficulties with Democratic interest groups, and claim in the end that these problems had forced him into the race.

Indeed, some of those who were working for the senator at the time said later that their greatest fear was that we would capitulate, adopt all his proposals, and then stand back while they died aborning in the Congress. They need not have worried. Although there were some in the Carter camp who were half-inclined to believe that we could stroke Teddy into not running, there was no possibility that the President would agree to support Kennedy's major positions.

As it developed, our response was to stick to our guns, but to try to do it in an accommodating way—a hybrid plan that proved to be predictably impotent.

My own view was that Kennedy would do everything he could to undermine the President, publicly and on the Hill, stopping just short of the point where his strategy would be too obvious to ignore. Given the general disinclination of the press to say anything unkind about him, he would have a lot of room to maneuver.

A review of coverage of the Carter-Kennedy conflict during the first nine or ten months of 1979 reveals little that can be remotely construed as critical of Kennedy on any score. There are numerous references to the "incompetence," "fumbling," "needlessly antagonistic," "controversial" Jimmy Carter. Kennedy, however, is portrayed as "committed" (to his convictions and his vision of the country and the party), "deeply troubled" (by Carter's apparent lack of concern for same), and "agonizing" (over whether duty and love of country compel him to seek the nomination).

If there was ever the slightest hint that calculation and ambition ever crossed the senator's mind or were ever absent from the President's, I never saw it then. Nor was I able to find it later.

* * *

My theory of the senator's behavior was solidified in the spring of 1979 by his reaction to the President's call for a windfall-profits tax on oil. We had anticipated his opposition to deregulation of oil prices, which the President had accomplished by executive action at the same time that he proposed the windfall tax. But a windfall tax was a different matter. He had been long and loudly in favor of such an idea.

Perhaps he would be content to demagogue decontrol and let it go at that? Not on your life. Immediately after the President's announcement, he was before the television cameras taking potshots, not at decontrol, but at the windfall tax. Never happen . . . bad strategy . . . no way the President could ever get it through Congress. He even suggested that it would divide the Democratic party and hurt the President's chances for renomination.

I suggested to reporters that these considerations never seemed to bother him with regard to national health insurance and other favorite pieces of legislation—with the usual lack of effect.

In the end, the windfall tax was passed early in 1980, without conspicuous help from Senator Kennedy. This was the behavior of a candidate, not a man worried about the issues that he had supported for a lifetime. That fact seemed obvious to those of us in the White House. If it occurred to those in the fourth estate, they were careful to keep it a secret from the public.

A few weeks before the windfall tax announcement, the tenth anniversary of Chappaquiddick came and went. Several news organizations, including the *Washington Post* and the *New York Times*, undertook major investigations to get at the truth of that incident. Not surprisingly, they were unable to come up with anything new.

The *Washington Post* gave witness to the kid-glove treatment generally accorded the senator by agreeing to an interview on Chappaquiddick in which the questions had to be presented in advance, and the senator and his staff retained the right to edit the responses before they were published. This arrangement raised eyebrows among politicians and journalists, including some of the latter at the *Post*.

"It was," said one *Post* reporter, "a total embarrassment. I never understood why you people [in the White House] never raised hell about it. If you had tried to set up that sort of thing for the President to talk about nuclear weapons, or Bert Lance to talk about his problem, or Billy Carter to talk about Libya, we would have laughed in your face, and then run an editorial crucifying you for even asking."

One reason we never raised hell about it was that we were at that time involved in the famous, or infamous, domestic policy summit at Camp David—the one that culminated in what came to be known as the malaise speech and in the firing of several Cabinet members. Suffice it to say for now that this story helped to divert public and press attention from the tenth-anniversary story.

As a result of all the above, the anniversary passed without much in the way of damaging publicity for Senator Kennedy. His people now say that this was a major factor in their decision to run. It led them to believe that the incident would not be a factor. It was a serious misjudgment.

The press had tried to find something new that would tell what actually happened. The thrust of the latest stories was that they could not find it, plus some speculation on the political impact of it all in case the senator sought the presidency. There were even a few polls that were interpreted as showing that most Americans were willing to "forgive and forget."

What was neglected was the fact that it is difficult for almost anyone who has ever taken the time to review the senator's actions and statements relating to that night to believe that he told the truth, or to doubt that he went to considerable trouble to cover up the truth. There are just too many inconsistencies and improbabilities.

The question that the press missed was similar to the one that brought down President Nixon. It is not whether the public is willing to forgive and forget a mistake, but whether the public is content to have as president a man who has consistently attempted to deceive them and cover up his own responsibility for the mistake. The public is willing to forgive, but not without being asked, and not in the face of repeated denials that there is anything much to be forgiven.

WILL
TEDDY RUN?

I n the late summer of 1979 we were treated to another piece of skillful gamesmanship by Senator Kennedy and another suspension of critical judgment by the press.

Leading up to Labor Day weekend, stories began to appear announcing a Kennedy family meeting at which the senator would ask the clan if he should make the race. Not since Sadat and Begin went to Camp David had a gathering received such a buildup.

Once the "meeting" was over, the details were immediately leaked. The print press was filled with heartrending accounts of the discussions that had taken place, complete with which family members had taken what positions and why. That night, CBS, that hard-hitting, no-nonsense news organization, led off the Cronkite show with a report, attributed to unidentified sources, that Senator Kennedy's wife and mother had said it was okay for him to run for president.

As it turned out, this rather questionable bit of news judgment came at the urging of Roger Mudd. He is an exceptional newsman, but also a longtime friend of the Kennedy family—a friendship that the Kennedys would terminate in exactly two months.

For a week you could hardly open a newspaper without running into a quote from a "Kennedy family intimate" describing the traumatic session. The stories particularly emphasized the concern for the effect of a race on the senator's wife, Joan. The fact that this concern had not noticeably affected the senator's behavior up to that point would certainly have been noted if any other politician had been involved.

There was hardly a journalist or a politician in Washington who had any doubt that the senator was running. Many say now that they considered the entire spectacle a charade. One does not normally leak word in advance of a meeting to discuss a "very private family decision" if it is truly intended to be private, or if there is any doubt about what the "decision" will be.

Even more to the point, Paul Kirk, the senator's chief political aide, has since revealed that the senator told him, before the meeting with the family, that he would definitely be in the race.

And if the point needs sharpening, Kennedy later denied that there had ever been any meeting where he had asked for an okay to run from anyone. What there had been, he said, was a series of discussions about the idea, and he had come away with the understanding that they would support whatever decision he made. Had all those "family intimates" been dreaming? Or had the Kennedy people put out a patently self-serving tale that made too good a story for any reporter to mess up by asking awkward questions, or implying the slightest touch of skepticism?

At the time, I tried to imagine the abuse and ridicule that would have descended upon our heads if we had attempted such a transparent bit of gimmickery. Jimmy Carter flying to Plains to confer with Miss Lillian, Billy, Ruth, and Gloria—plus assorted nieces, nephews, and cousins—on whether he should seek reelection. It made me shudder to think of it. We would have been up to our necks in cartoons and columns featuring Tobacco Road, Snopeses, and various other allusions to hillbillies and rednecks within two days.

There was, of course, a difference, as several reporters pointed out. The horrible tragedy of two Kennedy brothers still gripped and moved the nation. There was a reason for the senator to think about the feelings of his family as he made his decision, and I have no doubt that he did. But this highly advanced and publicized exercise was something else. At best, it was a staging for the cameras and the press of what may well have been an agonizing decision. In my admittedly cynical view, the carefully orchestrated exploitation of the emotions and sympathy of the nation only exacerbated the offense.

This incident had a more profound effect on my attitude toward Senator Kennedy than any other, before or since. Looking back on it years later, I have tried to convince myself that my judgment is too harsh, without success. The most I have been able to come up with is the grudging admission that I could be wrong, that perhaps there is some other reasonable explanation for it all. There may be, but I have not found it.

A part of my resentment results from the fact that I too was intimidated by the spectacle of it all. Although my feelings about it then were the same as they are now, I never could bring myself to suggest to a reporter, even privately, that we were merely watching a somewhat cynical play for public sympathy. It is not that I think it would have done much good. Knowing, as I do now, that many of them felt the same way, I find it hard to be too critical of them for not saying in public what I did not have the guts to say even in private.

The other thing that rankled about this incident was how starkly it contrasted to the treatment of Carter by the press. For at least a year, Carter's every statement and action had been analyzed in a political context. If he did something popular, he was pandering to public opinion. If he defied the popular mood, he was trying to combat his wishy-washy image by looking tough. If he defied Congress with a veto, he was preparing to run against a Congress controlled by his party, and blame it for his problems. If he compromised, it was a play for political backing in some key state.

Of course there were political considerations involved in almost every decision, as there have been for every president since George Washington. Whether the implication that this President almost never thought of anything else came through as strongly in print reporting as it seemed to me, others will have to judge. I can only say that reading back over the clips and the news summaries now is an even more disillusioning experience than it was at the time.

Whether journalists are generally too cynical about the motives of politicians is a separate question. In this case, "generally" does not apply. On the one hand you had a politician named James Earl Carter, who was treated primarily as a politician whether he was talking about Soviet aggression, nuclear war, energy, the budget, you name it. On the other, you had a politician named Edward Moore Kennedy, whose statements and actions were of interest primarily because he was about to be a candidate for the presidency, and who could count on almost anything he did or said being taken at face value.

To us this double standard seemed to apply to the interpretation of political events as well as to public statements.

In October the Florida Democratic party held caucuses to elect delegates to a party conference. As everyone had known for months, a straw poll on presidential preference was to be held at the same time. A group of Kennedy supporters, funded and encouraged by several unions closely allied with Kennedy, decided to challenge the President, and after several months of work held a press conference to announce that Kennedy would beat Carter by a substantial margin.

This, of course, drew a great deal of press attention, including some speculation that Carter might in fact lose among pundits who should have known better.

We did not need to have our attention directed to Florida. We had been watching it for some time. Sergio Bendixen and Mike Abrams, the organizers of the Kennedy campaign, had worked for Carter in 1976. We had since parted company over patronage and their feeling that Carter was too conservative. We knew them to be capable organizers, but incurable publicity hounds. (We also took some private satisfaction from the fact that Abrams's wife, who was an even better politician, had left him but stayed with the Carter camp.)

Their foolish prediction of victory and the press attention it attracted was just what we had been waiting for. We figured a sound trouncing might take some of the wind out of the Kennedy sails, at least shake the common assumption among Washington journalists that the nomination was his for the asking.

Wrong again. When the voting was over and Kennedy had indeed been soundly trounced, political analysts decided it really did not mean that much after all. It was no longer the "first test" or an "early indication of whether there is any support for Carter left anywhere." It was in retrospect just a misguided crusade by a couple of young, naïve Kennedy types that had actually taken place against the better judgment of the senator and his closest aides.

The fact that there had been consultation between the Florida operation and the senator's staff throughout was overlooked—the fact that this seemed to violate election laws (which prohibit coordination between such "independent" groups and the candidate they are supporting) and was directly in conflict with denials from the senator's office had been ignored from the start. Nor did the fact that members of the senator's family had gone down to campaign for him seem to make any difference.

The senator had lost, but he was clearly going to win the nomination anyway; therefore this contest had to be irrelevant. And so it was reported.

WHY IS TEDDY RUNNING?

Unbeknownst to any of us in the White House, a political event of the first magnitude was in the making during the summer of 1979. CBS had decided back in June to do an hour-long special on Edward M. Kennedy. (Apparently some CBS executives had about as little faith as I did in the sincerity of the senator's public agonizing.) They asked Roger Mudd to try to obtain an interview with Kennedy as part of the show. After some soul-searching—because of his close personal relationships with the Kennedys—Mudd agreed.

As envisioned by CBS, it should have been free campaign publicity. Crews were assigned to film the senator at work on Capitol Hill, camping with a host of Kennedy children, and relaxing with the family at Hyannis Port.

The media orgasm over the family "decision" did not hurt the project at all. Once that had occurred, the senator was covered as though he were a candidate, and the frenzied atmosphere around him was ideal for documentary footage. Here was the dutiful senator going about his job as the nation eagerly awaited his decision.

Of course the decision had already been made, but why not milk it a little? It suited Kennedy's purposes and the media's.

What turned a potential puff-piece into a political disaster was the interview—or interviews. There were actually two: the first in Hyannis Port on September 29 and the second in the senator's office on the Hill two weeks later. What Kennedy said, or did not say, in that interview has been analyzed to death. The result, as everyone now knows, was to raise the first doubts in the minds of Washington journalists that his nomination by acclamation would be assured as soon as he announced.

There are several things, however, about that interview that have particular bearing on a book about the press, and I will confine my comments to them.

The first point is that although you cannot find a journalist now who does not claim to have been shocked and profoundly affected by those interviews, there was precious little evidence of it in the reporting and analysis immediately following the airing of the special. There was a good deal of talk around town about how badly Kennedy had done, but not much "This raises questions about the man's qualifications" discussion, even in private. And almost no one could bring himself to raise that sort of issue in public.

On the whole, the analysis boiled down to "He was terrible, but he was tired," or "He wasn't prepared, poor staff work," or "He had a hard time answering questions about his candidacy since he hadn't officially announced," or "He hadn't taken the time to think those things through."

This last was particularly mind boggling since the things he supposedly hadn't had time to think through were what happened at Chappaquiddick and why he wanted to be President of the United States. It is certainly possible that the senator had not devoted sufficient time to how he wanted to phrase his responses to those questions, but it is highly likely that he knew very well how he wanted to handle those questions in general.

In fact, one does not have to be as cynical as this writer to see that as the most logical conclusion; his behavior for the next several months was perfectly consistent with his handling of those two questions in the Mudd interview.

The senator's subsequent behavior suggests that the decision had been made to stonewall on Chappaquiddick. Every answer in the CBS transcript on this subject was an obvious, albeit not very skillful, evasion. The one impression that comes through loud and clear is the determination not to add one new word to the record. When asked about inconsistencies in his previous statements and conflicts between those statements and physical evidence, the response was in effect "That's my story, and I'm sticking to it." And he has stuck to it until this very day.

The message in the "Why do you want to be President?" response was less apparent. But it would become obvious to anyone who cared to notice as soon as Senator Kennedy hit the campaign trail. The last thing he wanted to do was run a campaign based on his positions on the issues of the day. He was well to the left of the Democratic center, and he knew it. To have campaigned as himself would have endangered his chances at the nomination and destroyed any hope for a victory in the general election. Nor was he particularly anxious to get caught up in a discussion of what he would do that was different from what Carter had done.

Far better to talk about "leadership" and "releasing the native energy of the people" and kick hell out of your opponent in between. Comparing the senator's early campaign speeches with that first stumbling answer is like looking at the first and second drafts of the same text.

Senator Kennedy did not want to talk about what he stood for because it wouldn't sell, and because he thought Carter would collapse once he had declared opposition. If the senator continued to have some of the same problems in describing what he stood for in the months that followed, it was because his purpose was not to enlighten, but to obfuscate.

One of your all-time great pieces of conventional political wisdom is that, following the Mudd interview, poor Teddy got all the bad breaks. Carter, on the other hand, is commonly supposed to have been riding a wave of favorable publicity stemming from foreign policy crises in Iran and Afghanistan. How fortunate for Carter that he could sit in the White House, basking in the glow of all that favorable publicity, while Kennedy was getting his brains beaten out by "a relatively junior group of news reporters" who "seized on every fluff" and "magnified" the mistakes that are a part of every new campaign.

Some journalists were so offended by this terrible turn of events that they dashed off teary-eyed columns complaining about how unfair everyone, particularly the networks, was being.

Charles Seib, then the ombudsman for the *Washington Post*, wondered on November 22 if "the press [is] leaning over backwards to the point where it is now unfair to the man it was accused of favoring." In mid-December, Tom Shales, the television critic for the *Post*, in a column entitled (can you believe it?) "Teddy's Torment," and again on January 30 in "Petty for Teddy," accused the networks, and CBS in particular, of "seeking to destroy" the Kennedy candidacy.

Needless to say, neither Mr. Shales nor Mr. Seib expressed similar concern that the press might be getting a little carried away with their attacks on Carter.

More important, the whole thing was manufactured, cellophane-wrapped horse manure. The main thing that was bad about Teddy's press coverage was the contrast to the drooling adulation he had received since he first indicated a willingness to run against Carter. Compared to Carter, he was always treated like the second coming, and particularly by the networks.

There is no hard data available for November and December of 1979, but beginning with January of 1980, the data are there and the conclusions are hard to ignore.

In a book entitled *Over the Wire and on TV*,* Michael Robinson and Margaret Sheehan have rated press coverage as positive or negative for all the candidates, and then compiled a "press index" by comparing the percentage of positive and negative stories.

The only network rated was CBS, but Robinson and Sheehan cite evidence, including a ten-day sample of all three networks, that indicates that the positive/negative ratio of coverage for all three networks tended to be quite similar.

Their figures, which have predictably been ignored by those who were responsible for the coverage they call into question, are damning. They cause one to wonder exactly what it was that was so mightily offensive to Messrs. Seib and Shales.

From January until the end of the Democratic convention in August, Senator Kennedy's press index on CBS was just about a wash—slightly more positive than negative stories. Carter, that crafty manipulator of the press and the powers of the incumbency, had almost six negative stories for every one that was positive.

When journalists of the "poor Teddy" persuasion were shown these figures, they immediately claimed that they were only talking

*New York: Russell Sage Foundation, 1983.

about the first few months of the campaign, before the Iran situation began to go sour. That was when Teddy was so ill used.

Well, what about the first few months? In January on CBS Kennedy had a −28, but Carter was at −31. In February it was Kennedy, −12; Carter, −9. In March it was −28 for both. And in April, it was Kennedy, −23; Carter, −51. Cumulatively for the first four months, the comparison was Carter down 3, even, even, Carter down 28.

When confronted with this information, distinguished analysts began to mutter darkly about methodology, and who did the rating, and press secretaries writing "get even" books.

On UPI, the print organization chosen by Robinson and Sheehan, the ratings were more favorable to Carter, but hardly evidence of a "get Teddy" conspiracy. For the first four months, Kennedy's press was slightly more negative than Carter's. Through August Kennedy came out slightly on the positive side, and Carter was dead even.

In Carter's case, Robinson and Sheehan say, his press was even worse than the figures show. Which is hard for even me to believe. How much worse can you get than terrible?

Most of the stories were rated as ambiguous for all candidates. Only those seen as positive or negative by all the judges who did the ratings were so scored. But fully 90 percent of the "ambiguous" stories about Carter were "shaded toward unfavorable." (A majority considered them negative, but not all.)

Of course, Robinson and Sheehan do not attempt to measure degrees of negativism. Although that is a highly subjective bit of business, you cannot really argue with the fact that there is a real and important difference between saying that a candidate has simply made a mistake and saying that he has revealed a basic flaw in character. As a matter of fact, if you have a candidate like Kennedy, whose eyes tend to roll anytime the word "character" is mentioned, it might be considered a great favor for every shortcoming to be portrayed as an honest error.

From the White House, that is just what seemed to be happening, more often than not, for the entire eight months of the primary campaign. If Carter exaggerated, as he was wont to do, it was a sure sign of a devious mind. In Kennedy's case, it was because he did not have his stump speech together quite yet.

Kennedy's transgressions were misdemeanors. Carter's were hanging offenses.

One early example of this tendency to give Kennedy the benefit of every doubt, and Carter the doubt of every benefit, occurred during the early days of the campaign year. It complemented the alibi that the senator's early stumbling was the result of routine start-up problems, rather than the innate difficulties of trying to run against an incumbent President without ever saying specifically what you would do differently.

This theory, which persists to this day, holds that it was Iran and the taking of the hostages, or Iran plus the invasion of Afghanistan, that laid poor Teddy low and saved that rascal Carter. We shall never know what would have happened in 1980 without either of those two international crises, but there is evidence that Teddy's coronation might not have been a sure thing.

For the first eight months of 1979, Kennedy enjoyed a comfortable lead over Carter. This was the period when the press was helping to maintain the fiction that he was a noncandidate who would never run unless it was necessary to save the country. But the Labor Day weekend family meeting put an end to that game. Voters began to assess the senator as a potential President rather than a convenient vehicle for protest. And his standing in the polls began to drop. From September through early October, Kennedy's margin declined by 40 percent.

After his loss in the Florida straw vote in October, the senator blithely declared that it did not mean anything anyway, and "the first real test" was Iowa. The press, who had been reporting Florida as "the first real test" until Kennedy lost, mumbled apologies for their stupidity, snuggled into his lap, and agreed that he was right as usual.

Less than three weeks later, as our embassy in Tehran was being overrun and the day before the Mudd interview was aired, Carter beat Kennedy by better than two to one in a poll at the Iowa Jefferson-Jackson Day Dinner. The gathering should have been an opportunity for Kennedy, who was always strongest among the more active party members. Nor had the senator failed to make an effort, sending Ethel Kennedy and her son Joe to represent him at the meeting.

Instead it turned out to be a clear signal that the senator's warts were becoming visible to the people of the country, if not to his Washington claque, even before Iran and Mudd. When the official caucus vote took place almost three months later, the Carter margin of victory was roughly the same as it had been at the dinner.

Kennedy then decided to change his campaign style. His vague promises to restore leadership without describing what he would do differently were not selling. In the course of three days he came up with a completely different set of campaign themes and proposals, some of which happened to be in direct conflict with what he had been saying for the past three months.

The new Kennedy emerged on January 28, one week after the Iowa caucuses, in a speech at Georgetown University in Washington and in a follow-up address at Harvard two weeks later. We, not surprisingly, considered the speeches to be demagoguery of the first order. The senator warned that Carter's "failed foreign policy" was leading us into war. He held up visions of "a nightly television body count of America's children." Shamelessly exploiting the resistance to any form of military service for which Harvard has become famous, he declared his principled opposition to "spill[ing] American blood in order to top off gas tanks here at home." If the Russians launched an invasion of Saudi Arabia, the proper American response, according to Teddy, was not to fight, but to buy Volkswagens. To make sure no one missed his point, he declared that both the taking of the hostages in Iran and the Soviet invasion of Afghanistan had been Carter's fault.

I was both angry and overjoyed when I heard the speeches. The next day I began to refer reporters to the dates and places where Kennedy had warmly supported, only a few weeks earlier, the "bloody" policies he now condemned. I pointed out that he had supported a firm response to the invasion of Afghanistan while campaigning in Iowa, and had seen the light just in time to recruit volunteers from the college campuses of the Northeast. When that produced not one story on this remarkable transformation, I photocopied articles from Iowa papers with his tough-on-the-Russians rhetoric and offered them to journalists to compare with his Georgetown and Harvard speeches.

One such incident that sticks in my mind followed a particularly tough piece on Carter by NBC's political correspondent Tom Petit. I called him to suggest that he take a look at the rather striking contrast between the old and the new Kennedy, and quoted the earlier statements to him. "Very interesting," he said, "need to do something on that." Would I send the news clips to him? Of course I did, and of course nothing came of it. Petit said later that he had gotten tied up with something else and never got back to the story.

Apparently a lot of journalists found themselves terribly busy with other things when the opportunity arose to examine the senator's inconsistencies.

What most of them were busy doing was kicking Carter's teeth in every time he opened his mouth, particularly if he said anything critical of Kennedy. The record of those first few months is not open to dispute. Almost every step taken by Carter to respond to Soviet aggression was politically dangerous, if not downright unpopular, from the grain embargo to draft registration. In each case, Kennedy waved the bloody shirt and attacked the President's proposals. (That is actually an oversimplification. He only attacked the grain embargo in Iowa, waiting until he got to the Ivy League campuses and the New England primaries to attack draft registration.)

When the President or Vice-President had the temerity to suggest that the senator might be playing a little politics with national security or taking the easy way out, it was Carter and Mondale who were attacked as demagogues and opportunists.

At this point, I should make it clear that the decidedly uneven nature of the press coverage up to this point was not solely the product of the cuddly relationship between Kennedy and the Washington press corps. Another major and separate factor was an intense and growing dislike of Carter.

The reasons for this antipathy are still difficult to completely understand, at least for me. But there is no doubt that it existed. The several dozen reporters I have interviewed for this book were almost unanimous in listing a personal distaste for Carter, on the part of either themselves or their colleagues, as a factor in how he was treated by the press.

The most common reason cited was "He didn't understand

us," or more pointedly "He didn't like us." We shall pass quickly over the question of whether grown men and women who are supposed to be professionals should have to be liked and understood in order to do their job properly. The answer is that they should not, but they do.

Another frequently mentioned complaint was that they, the reporters, did not understand Carter. There is some truth to that, although my interpretation of it may differ drastically from that of some of those who made the comment.

For most journalists, Carter was different—not only from most politicians and Presidents they had covered, but from them. He was a small-town Southern Baptist with a set of values and beliefs that made many of them decidedly uncomfortable.

It was not so much his outward signs of religion that pained the press. They were accustomed to and reasonably tolerant of hypocrites. As at least three of them later would say, in separate interviews: "The problem with Carter was that we knew he meant it"—or words to that effect.

Most journalists are convinced that no one makes it very far in politics without selling a sizable chunk of his soul. But here was a guy who not only claimed to have done it differently, but who was clearly of the opinion that politics as usual was wrong. To make things even worse, this guy was setting himself up to be not only better than most politicians, but also better than most journalists. There was an implicit challenge involved, or at least many journalists thought there was, to prove that Carter was at least as rotten as all the rest.

The sad fact is that many political reporters are a good bit more familiar and comfortable with politicians who lie, cheat, and steal than with one who prays—particularly if he prays in private and with conviction.

Carter did not fit the mold in other ways. He was a southerner. This did not endear him to some. Jack Nelson, Washington bureau chief for the *Los Angeles Times*, recalls a colleague from the *Boston Globe* delivering himself of his views on the subject just as Carter began to emerge from the pack in the 1976 campaign: "This guy Carter may win the nomination and he may even make the best President of the bunch, but he is a redneck, Baptist, Bible thumper and I don't like it one damn bit."

What was more, Carter did not fit the southern-pol stereo-type, which was unforgivable. Not only did he practice as well as preach his religion, he did not tell racist jokes, even in private, and he did not drink large quantities of bourbon and pat strange women on the fanny. Lastly, he did not particularly enjoy bullshit sessions with the boys.

Even his political views fit none of the standard journalistic molds for southerners. He certainly was not a rehabilitated segregationist, but neither was he one of those knee-jerk, professional southern liberals who delight in entertaining Yankees with drunken expositions on the dark and mysteriously evil soul of the Southland. Nor was he one of the new country-club southern Republicans who had moved from the farm to the suburbs, bought a station wagon, become an Episcopalian, and learned to tell jokes about rednecks as well as blacks.

Carter had, heaven forbid, gotten the vast majority of the black vote against certified Washington-type liberals in 1976, and he was doing the same thing against Teddy Kennedy in 1980. So this guy was obviously weird and probably devious. He had to be watched carefully.

There was another irritant in the relationship. Carter was smarter than most reporters and clearly knew it. Reporters are not, whatever their other faults may be, stupid. In fact, they take pride in being intellectually, as well as morally, superior to most of the people they cover. They do not take kindly to being looked down upon by any politician, particularly not a peanut farmer from some piddly-ass little gnat-hole in south Georgia.

Finally, Carter did not work at being lovable. He did his job and expected everyone else, including journalists, to do theirs, without a great deal of petting and stroking. He did not particularly like having slanderous things said about him and his associates, and he did not see any reason to pretend that he thought those responsible were great Americans doing a wonderful job.

To a degree, Jimmy Carter's problems with the press were symptomatic of his difficulties with other parts of official Washington. None of that semipermanent crowd of journalists, lobbyists, and bureaucrats knew Jimmy Carter when he moved into the White House. Few of them knew him much better when he left. Part of it was nobody's fault. He was never a Washington figure until inauguration day and there had never been an opportunity for personal relationships to develop.

Jimmy Carter lacked, to a greater extent than any other modern President, a loyal coterie of friends and die-hard supporters among those people who remain permanently in Washington as administrations come and go. Once a man becomes President, making new friends is a difficult undertaking. There are few people, even in Washington, who can forget they are talking to a President and be enough of themselves for a true friendship to develop. There are even fewer with whom a President could afford to drop his guard and be himself.

However, I must say in all honesty that one of my great regrets is that I did not make a greater effort to get the President together socially with small groups of journalists—not the White House correspondents, who are fearful of becoming too close to a President and probably with good reason, but editors, columnists, and some of the senior network people.

In 1979, Jerry Rafshoon began to set up a series of small dinners with these types, and it did help some. I am convinced that had we started in February of 1977, our relationships with the fourth estate would have been better. They certainly could not have been much worse.

FROM BAD
TO AWFUL_____

If the attitude of the press toward Jimmy Carter was bad during the first half of the 1980 primary campaign, it turned terrible during the first week in April. That week, and the week that preceded it, marked the collapse of our final effort to negotiate the release of the hostages through what has come to be known as the French Connection, and the collapse of the last vestiges of restraint by the press in coming down on Carter with both feet.

If there is one thing that White House press staff and White House press agree upon, it is that the events from Saturday, March 29, through the middle of the next week were the final blow to our hopes of reestablishing a decent relationship with the press. From that point forward, the Carter administration was damaged goods. The idea that we were devious, and not above playing politics with the lives of the hostages, became part of the conventional wisdom for many who were covering us. Nothing we could do or say would change their minds.

The first "agreement" with Iran had collapsed in mid-March with the failure of what passed for an Iranian government to live up to its commitments to us and to the United Nations commission.

After serious consideration and partially as a result of the pleading of our intermediaries, the President had agreed to try to revive the negotiating process that produced the original agreement. On March 25, the President met personally with Christian Bourget, one of those intermediaries, and gave him a brief personal note to be used as Bourget saw fit. It outlined the fundamental U.S. position:

- Release of our diplomats

- U.S. recognition of the results of the Iranian revolution and normal relations with the new government

- The right for Iran to air whatever grievances it had at an appropriate international forum

At the same time, to make sure there was no misunderstanding, the President decided it would be wise to let the Iranian authorities know in no uncertain terms that if they reneged again, the consequences would be severe. Plans for a rescue operation had been formulated, and though no one ever said so in my presence, there was a feeling that if this effort failed, some sort of military operation would almost certainly be the next step.

He dispatched a message to Iranian President Abolhassan Bani-Sadr making it clear that if the hostages had not been transferred to government control by April 1 (as had been agreed upon), we would be forced to consider our diplomatic efforts to obtain their release a failure. It was a threat, and a not very thinly veiled one at that.

In the early hours of Saturday morning, March 29, I was awakened by a call from the press office duty officer. There was, he said, a story moving out of Iran about a letter from Carter to Khomeini in which the President had apologized for American sins against the Iranian people in the most abject terms. The bogus message went on to say that the President understood "that the occupation of our embassy . . . could have been regarded as a reasonable action."

The press office was being flooded with calls for confirmation and additional information. I told the duty officer he could categorically deny that any such letter had been sent by any American official, but to go no further than that. I would be down shortly.

I called Hamilton to let him know what was up. Then I checked with the State Department duty officer, to make sure they had seen the same report. They had. After a quick shower I set off for the White House, less than a fifteen-minute drive at that hour of the morning.

On the way in the thought occurred to me that maybe there was something going on that I did not know about. I had stayed very close to the hostage negotiations on almost a daily basis. A letter like that would have been totally inconsistent with everything we were doing. But still, maybe we had sent something that the Iranians had rewritten or quoted out of context. But even out of context the words and phrases in the story could not have come from any American official in his right mind, much less the President.

Hamilton was in his office shortly after I arrived, and he laid my concerns about the existence of another letter to rest immediately. I went back to assure the press, who by that time were roosting in the lampshades of my office, that the reported letter was a fabrication.

They were, to say the least, skeptical. And this time I did not blame them. The whole thing did not make sense to them or to me. A few of them thought I had been sent out to lie to provide a cover for some murky diplomatic maneuvering. Those who were more kindly disposed thought I was being misled by someone else in the government. Everyone was sure that there was more to this than met the eye. Indeed there was.

We were in an awkward situation. So far my conversations with White House reporters had been brief. I had been able to get by with the flat denial I had given the duty officer: the letter, or message, or whatever it was, was a fabrication.

Sooner or later, once the reporters had filed those first reactions and gotten the sleep out of their eyes and their wits about them, they would realize that there might be more to this thing. They would then want to know exactly what that more was. And we were in no position to satisfy their curiosity.

In the first place, we honestly did not know where the fake message had come from, although we were beginning to have some suspicions. It sounded very much as though it had been a well-intentioned but ill-conceived effort by our intermediaries to improve the climate in Tehran. We could hardly say such a thing, however. In the first place, it was only conjecture at that point. More important, it would have destroyed the effectiveness of our only regular contacts with any Iranian officials.

Beyond that, the last thing we wanted was for the President's ultimatum to become public, thus forcing Bani-Sadr and the crazies who were running the country into an even more defiant posture. If I admitted that there was another message, a journalistic manhunt would begin to find someone who would tell reporters what the message said; and if past experience was any guide, they might well find someone in the American government who was stupid enough to tell them.

Even if they did not, for me to admit that there was a message, claim that it did not say what had been reported, and then refuse to reveal anything about what it did say would make our credibility problems even worse.

After a rather unpleasant session with the President, in which he freely expressed his opinion of reporters who would believe some anonymous Iranian official instead of the President of the United States, we decided that I had to have a sit-down session with the press and try to convince them I was telling the truth.

I called the reporters into my office instead of going to the briefing room. The more informal office setting seemed to work better for dealing with complicated matters. There was less baiting and fewer interruptions. I essentially repeated the original statement in as many ways as I could:

- "No such message has been sent to anyone anywhere by the President or anyone else in this government."

- "I can tell you with absolute assurance that this thing is a fake. I don't know where it came from, but it didn't come from this government."

- "You've read this thing. Do you really believe that the President or anyone else in the government would use the words contained in it?"

I even cited Teddy Kennedy, of all people, for support, reminding the press that in December, Tehran radio and newspapers had reported a supposed message from Kennedy to Khomeini asking for a meeting and stating that the senator was prepared "to spill his blood" in the service of the Iranian revolution. That message had, of course, been a fake, I said, and this one was too.

The briefing actually turned out better than I had expected. With a fair amount of wriggling and squirming, I managed to avoid a direct answer to the "Were any messages sent?" question. I also avoided being so obvious in my evasion that the curiosity of the reporters was aroused.

In an attempt to make sure that my on-the-record comments were precisely understood, a background briefing was arranged at the State Department at which reporters were informed that there had indeed been an exchange of ideas between the two governments and that some of the purported message was "not inconsistent" with some of those ideas.

Feeling that the best had been made of a bad situation, I left to make a speech that evening in Columbus to the Ohio Jefferson-Jackson Day Dinner. I should have recognized the ominous portent when the centerpiece of the buffet table—a four-foot-high ice carving of a donkey—collapsed into the canapés as I was two minutes into my opening remarks.

The next morning as I was showering in a Columbus motel, the Iranians—for reasons known only to themselves—revealed the threat message. And a large number of reporters, for reasons known only to themselves, were deeply offended that neither I nor the State Department had given them any hint that another message existed.

I saw no reason why they should feel that I was obligated to send them scurrying after a message that might well prove extremely harmful if they found it. I had said "no such message" repeatedly. And although some of the reporters had missed the importance of the word "such," both the *New York Times* and the *Washington Post* had carefully included it in their accounts. (Strangely, although the *Times* had at first quoted me correctly, two days later they were claiming in another story that I had said "no" messages of any kind were sent.)

I believe now as I did then that my comments and those at State were honest and proper under the circumstances.

But what I believed was beside the point. The reporters had missed a story, and they had decided to make us pay for it.

What was worse, some journalists used the no-letter–no-such-letter squabble as a basis to suggest that maybe Carter or someone else in the administration had indeed sent something like the apology to someone in Iran.

Others had to reach even further to get their licks in. One of the strangest was a column by Rowland Evans and Robert Novak, two bombastic rascals whose only redeeming virtue is their lack of pretension to being anything else (except for Evans every now and then). This time they outdid themselves. Their argument was that even though nobody actually thought Carter had sent such a message, there were a lot of people who thought this was just the sort of message he would have sent if he had sent one. Furthermore, the fact that people were thinking that was an even stronger indictment of Carter than if he had actually sent the message. So there!

The few "facts" contained in the column were as unfactual as the reasoning was perverted. In October this dynamic duo would top even this performance with another column on Iran, but more on that later.

While Novak (semi-affectionately known as the Prince of Darkness) and Evans (not affectionately known as anything by anybody, including Novak) were revving up for their column, I was on my way to Milwaukee. At the request of our state coordinator, I had agreed to stop by on the way back from Ohio. The Wisconsin primary was to be held in two days, and although we appeared to be in good shape, there was no need to take any chances. When the trip was scheduled several days earlier, the purpose was to "give us a presence in the state" on the weekend before the primary. Now we would have a presence, even though we did not need it. But hardly the kind we wanted.

I struggled through a press conference that was, predictably, devoted entirely to the message fiasco. To make matters worse, those in attendance were either local reporters, with only a vague idea of what had been happening over the past few days, or national political correspondents, who had spent the past several days out of Washington and had only a little better feel for the nuances of the two briefings that had been held the day before.

When I got to Washington that night, the President was so concerned about the press reaction that he asked me to call a group of bureau chiefs into the White House so he could talk to them on an off-the-record basis. He was irritated about their doubting our word, and they were upset that we had not tipped them off about the other message. Most of all, he was concerned about the credibility problem that had developed. He wanted to try to set the record straight.

It was a good session. He explained what had happened on the messages, at least as far as he could without knowing who had fabricated the apology letter or why, or what had prompted the Iranians to release the threat letter. He also explained to them that we were nearing the end of a delicate set of negotiations that he hoped would bring about the release of our hostages, or at least their transfer from the hands of the militants who had invaded the embassy to the control of the government.

It was the second successful briefing in two days—or so we thought. But it too would come back to haunt us.

On that day, Sunday, and on Monday, we received messages from our intermediaries and one from Bani-Sadr himself that the deal had been cut. A majority of the Revolutionary Council had approved the transfer of the hostages. Bani-Sadr would announce the decision in a speech at noon on Tuesday, Iranian time. (The first messages actually predicted a Monday announcement. We were later told that there had been a delay, but that everything was still on track.)

Tuesday was also the day of the Wisconsin primary. It was important to us, because we had lost badly to Kennedy in New York the week before, after a humiliating mix-up in communications on a UN vote. But constant polling over the weekend had substantially relieved our concerns. Pat Caddell, one of the world's great pessimists, was predicting a big victory. His last run of numbers on Sunday showed Carter with a solid 15-point lead that could go as high as 25.

We gathered in the Oval Office in the early hours of Tuesday morning to await the first reports on Bani-Sadr's speech. It would require a response of some sort. A message from Iranian Foreign Minister Sadegh Ghotbzadeh on Monday had specifically requested that the President acknowledge the announcement as a "constructive step."

The primary in Wisconsin was far from our minds as we waited for the first wire service reports to come in, since we had no diplomats in positions who could cable us a report. As things turned out, we would have been better off to have given at least some thought to the political events of the day, and to the bitter cynicism with which the press viewed the President's every action.

When the first English translation of Bani-Sadr's speech was received, about 5:30 A.M., it was almost, but not quite, what we were looking for. It promised to transfer the hostages, but there were conditions. The most troublesome was the last. It demanded that we recognize the right of the Majlis, the Iranian parliament, to decide the fate of the hostages. This was not acceptable. The words "Iranian parliament" were a contradiction in terms. We could not be in a position of appearing to give advance approval to whatever this yet-to-be-convened legislative assemblage of a seriously unstable government might decide to do.

In the end, however, we agreed that we had no choice but to respond positively. If we said nothing, or responded negatively, the arrangement would certainly collapse. We would react positively, announce a hold on additional sanctions, attempt to finesse the Majlis question with a comment about the competence of the institution to deal with the question, and hope for the best.

We also agreed unanimously that the President's response should not be delayed. It was now approaching midafternoon in Iran. Knowing the fragile nature of all agreements in that country, we did not want to let the situation sit overnight.

A presidential statement was agreed upon. I asked, without giving the question much thought, whether the President would prefer to go to the briefing room or invite the press into the Oval Office. He said it would be all right to bring them into his office. That suited me fine, since the network correspondents had said just a few minutes earlier that the Oval Office would be their preference.

At 7:20 A.M. the President made his statement, a few questions were asked, and the press scurried out to file their stories.

Later, some would accuse the President of injecting too much optimism into his comments, of hyping his reaction beyond what the facts would support. That charge simply will not stand up to a reading of the transcript of what he actually said. He stated clearly that we had no reason to expect that the hostages would actually be transferred except for Bani-Sadr's statement. This was actually an understatement, as those who had attended the Sunday evening off-the-record session knew, because we had in fact received private assurances prior to Bani-Sadr's speech.

Others pointed to the fact that the statements had been made from the Oval Office as proof that we were trying to make a bigger story out of it. But I have found no one who is willing to say that he or she would have treated it any differently had it been made in the briefing room, which was the other option.

The reason for the recriminations by the press was that it soon became obvious that the Iranians had again failed to keep their word. Although Bani-Sadr himself had termed the response on the Majlis adequate two days after it was made, the excuse given later was that it was inadequate.

Almost immediately, Senator Kennedy accused the President of manipulating news from Iran to help us with the Wisconsin primary—which, by the way, we had won by a landslide, and with almost exactly the same margin that Caddell had been predicting for almost a week. The press took up Kennedy's attack and went at Carter tooth and tong. Here was absolute proof that the President was the devious, manipulative bastard they had always thought he was. They were, by God, determined to make sure the country knew about it.

The *New York Times* front-paged a story headed IRAN'S SHADOW ON THE PRIMARY. It was a masterpiece of innuendo. And it was one of those stories that I strongly suspected contained manufactured quotes. According to this story, Carter "aides conceded" that the timing of his early morning statement "was designed for maximum impact in the primary states." Certainly no aide who had been in the meeting said such a thing. Indeed, they have all, to a person, said just the opposite. I had personally and repeatedly denied that this was a factor, explaining that the timing was dictated by events in Iran. The *Times* totally ignored the denials and the explanation.

Declaring that "the President's handling of the crisis has finally emerged as a full-fledged issue in the campaign" (which must have pleased Teddy), the *Times* cited Carter's off-the-record meeting with senior news executives on Sunday evening as evidence of his politicization of the crisis. Carter's concern that some American journalists were putting as much credence in statements from

Iranian crazies as in statements from the White House had to be politically motivated.

The *Times* continued to play games with the "no such message" issue, this time using the correct quote but implying that there was somehow a contradiction in saying that no such message as the apology had been sent, when other messages, decidedly different in tone and substance, had been sent.

The *Washington Post* story was even worse. In fact, it was the absolute worst performance by two normally responsible reporters in the entire four years of the Carter administration. To make sure no one mistook their editorial position, their front-page "news analysis" was entitled DIPLOMACY AS POLITICS.

I knew we were in for it when the story opened by stating that Carter's day had begun "shortly after seven in the morning, as the voters in Wisconsin and Kansas started going to the polls." Every reporter on the White House beat knew by then that the President's day had actually begun about three-thirty, when he arose to dress and begin the anxious wait for what Bani-Sadr's speech would say. But to have mentioned that might have confused the reader, who was supposed to believe that Carter had spent his whole day thinking about politics and primaries, not hostages.

As for the President's statement, it "was more an exercise in domestic politics than international diplomacy." It was likened to President Nixon's "Peace is at hand" statement before the 1972 elections. (The statement was actually made by Kissinger, but why compare Carter with Kissinger when you can hang Nixon around his neck?)

"The timing [of the statement] was meant to coincide with the early morning television news programs."

The jump page was headed CARTER VICTORIES ABETTED BY OVAL OFFICE TELEVISION, a claim for which there was not and never has been one ounce of support.

According to the *Post*, those of us who met in the Oval Office that morning were facing the "political problem of how to get the optimistic news to the voters before they went to the polls." We were concerned because our "political operatives . . . sensed a growing erosion in the President's support" in Wisconsin. Our polls, and those of the news organizations, were in fact showing just the opposite.

Each one of these *Post* statements was demonstrably false. Those who wrote and disseminated the statements were well aware they were false. Their publication as fact on the front page of the *Washington Post* was incredibly damaging because they set the tone for the treatment of the President that was to continue throughout the campaign and beyond. (The *Post* also cited, as yet another example of Carter's low cunning, an attack on the idea of wage and price controls before the AFL-CIO convention. Less biased observers not caught up in a feeding frenzy might have given the President credit for political courage, since labor had come out in favor of wage and price controls.)

Rereading that amazing collection of error, smear, and fantasy almost three years later, I find it as infuriating now as it was at the time. It speaks volumes about much that is wrong with journalism.

In the first place, it pretends to tell readers things that the journalists could not possibly know. All the categorical statements on why we did what we did, the purpose of the President's statement, the role of timing, and so on, fall into that category.

It is one thing for a reporter to say that according to someone who was involved in a decision, the reasons for it were this or that or the other. It is quite another thing to baldly impute motivations to a President of the United States, or anyone else for that matter, based entirely on a hunch, or more likely, in this case, what a reporter wishes to believe. That sort of writing belongs in historical novels, not in a responsible newspaper.

The offense is aggravated when the reporter's musings are directly contradicted by all those who are in a position to know what has happened. As they were in this case.

This sort of journalism is, unfortunately, more typical of the *Post* than other major news organizations. It seems to be a part of the desire to project an image of always being on the inside. Perhaps it is a result of the additional pressure that comes from being the hometown paper. Whatever the reason, the result in this case was that not having been on the inside, and not knowing what had gone on, the reporters made it up.

Making up blind quotes to support your thesis (as I suspected the *Times* of doing) is bad enough. Making up reasons and motivations is infinitely worse. The *Times* quote from an anonymous aide was still presented as one person's opinion, although the implication was that the person was in a position to know. The treatment in the *Post* was a long compilation of absolutely false and tremendously damaging allegations, all stated as fact.

(To be absolutely fair to the *Post*, opposing views were not completely neglected. In their thirty-paragraph diatribe, all the denials, explanations, and counterarguments that I and other administration officials had presented received nine words.)

It is perhaps understandable that the two reporters who produced the piece could get caught up in the frustrations of trying to cover a difficult and complex matter and swept along by the emotionalism of their comrades. We all get carried away and do regrettable things on occasion. What defies comprehension, however, is that any sane editor could have put such a thing on the front page.

Unfortunately for us, the upper echelons of the *Post* were just as caught up in the "Carter is a conniving creep" mentality as their reporters. To make matters worse, the higher-ups were unencumbered by any factual information whatsoever, except for the President's vain attempt to explain what was really happening on the previous Sunday evening.

Some journalists apparently thought Senator Kennedy's alibi for his landslide losses in Wisconsin and Kansas had been too modest, and the press's brief on his behalf too limited. A few days after Kennedy blamed his defeat on the President's manipulation of the hostage crisis, *Washington Post* columnist David Broder decided, upon reflection, that all of Teddy's losses for the past month and a half were probably a result of Carter's sly manipulation of the media and foreign policy.

Mr. Broder's attitude toward Jimmy Carter had not been what one would call positive since before he was elected. He was offended by Carter's 1976 campaign against "Washington insiders" and never seemed to quite get over it.

His private opinions were reportedly even harsher than those he expressed in print. In fact, many of the criticisms he expressed were valid, at least in part. My chief complaint with David Broder had not been that his criticisms were unfair, but that it seemed strange that he had almost never been able to find anything that Carter did right that was worth mentioning. His approach to the Carter administration seemed to be "If you can't find something bad to say, don't say anything."

In this particular instance, however, Mr. Broder outdid himself. He first pointed out to the *Post*'s readers—who must have been deeply shocked by the revelation—that the President had actually stooped so low as to grant interviews to local newspapers and television stations in the weeks before primaries were held. To make matters worse, these interviews were "self-serving." Presumably, they were in contrast to the interviews and statements from Senator Kennedy, which were always selflessly complimentary to his opponent and modestly deprecating of his own talents and qualifications.

But then comes the meat of the column: Carter has also been making news just prior to every primary. Would you believe that every action that Carter has taken on foreign or domestic affairs has come within a few days of a primary or caucus for the past eleven weeks? Would you also believe that there has been a primary or caucus every week for the past eleven weeks?

As Mr. Broder well knew, any action the President took from mid-January on would inevitably fall within the suspicion of occurring only a "few days before an important primary." Moreover, Broder also knew that the President had little or no control over the timing of many of these "managed" news events. Most were reactions to external developments.

Others were "media events" we had tried desperately to keep secret: a trip by Hamilton Jordan to Panama to try to work out serious differences between the Shah and his new hosts, and stories in early March about the first agreement to bring about the release of the hostages. (On this last item, Broder went so far as to imply that the President might have been less than candid when he stated that the Iranians had reneged on the deal, which was a rather surprising insinuation inasmuch as the UN delegation that had taken part in those deliberations said exactly the same thing in even stronger terms before the President said it.)

It was, in my view, one of the tackier bits of journalism. And the fact that it had come from Broder, who has a reputation for being restrained, made the effect that much worse. But one should not be too hard on David Broder; the pack was in full cry. If you want to be a trendsetter, you have to stay out front.

Broder was certainly in step with his colleagues. At about the same time, Lesley Stahl of CBS came out with the movie version of his column, complete with pictorial evidence of Carter "making news just prior to every primary." Though Broder had not asked our reaction to his allegations, Lesley did. She simply chose to ignore my observation that any day in the past two months would have been just prior to a primary or caucus plus all other explanations for why things happened when they did that failed to support her indictment.

From our side it was like spitting into a hurricane. I pointed out to reporters that both their polls and our own had shown that we had Wisconsin won many days before Tuesday. That the timing had been determined by events in Tehran. That an immediate presidential response had been part of the agreement. That some of them, particularly CBS, had reported from sources in Tehran that the hostages would be transferred *before* the President made his statement.

I even suggested that they consider for a moment what every political analyst knows: that statements made on election eve seldom influence votes. And this news had come even later, on election morning, too late to make the morning papers. The only Wisconsin voters who would even have known about it before they voted were the roughly 10 percent that watched the morning news, or the few others who might have heard about it on the radio or seen it in an evening paper before voting.

It was all to no avail; the judgment had been made and there was no changing it.

Carter's press index on CBS as computed by Robinson and Sheehan dropped to a −51 for the month of April. Carter would get more negative than positive stories every month for the rest of the campaign. In other words, "There was almost no 'good news' about Carter whatever on 'Evening News.'" To make matters worse, the negative stories would have a cutting edge to them that was lacking in the coverage of other candidates. A significant portion of those reporting the race had simply written Jimmy Carter off. As far as they were concerned, he deserved the worst they could do to him. They could, and would, do a lot to him before they were through.

THE RIGHT TO LIE_____

S ince the day the first reporter asked the first tough question of a government official, there has been an ongoing debate about whether government has the right to lie.

The debate took on its present form one day in 1963, when then Pentagon spokesman Arthur Sylvester, for reasons known only to himself, responded to the question officially and honestly. "Yes," he said, "under certain circumstances I think government does have the right to lie."

The resulting furor has made every sitting press secretary and senior government official leery of the question from that day since. Like all my predecessors, I was always careful not to give a direct response. It was one of those questions for which you prepare and keep on file a standard evasion.

But Sylvester, of course, was right. In certain circumstances, government has not only the right but a positive obligation to lie. For me, that right-obligation flows directly from two other principles:

First, that government has a legitimate right to secrecy in certain matters because the welfare of the nation requires it. In other cases, individuals, even public figures, have a certain right to privacy because common decency demands it.

Secondly, the press has a right to print what it knows within very broad limits, without prior restraint, because the survival of democratic government depends on it.

Those two principles are often in conflict. Fortunately, the confrontation is not usually irreconcilable. Questions can be evaded. Answers can be devised that may mislead, but do not directly misrepresent. A "no comment" can sometimes be used without its being taken as a confirmation. Or the reporter can be sworn to secrecy himself and told why it is that certain information would be terribly damaging if published.

That is usually the case, but not always. Occasionally, the conflict is so sharp and the matter involved so important that there is no way to slide off the point. There is simply no answer that is both true and responsible. In such cases, the only decent thing to do is to lie and, I would argue, to make it the most convincing lie you can devise.

In my four years in the White House, I was only faced with that type of situation twice.

The first involved a question from a so-called reporter who was noted for trading in gossip and personal scandal, and who worked for a publication that had an even worse reputation in that regard.

The question involved the personal life of a colleague and that of his family. To have responded with what I believed to be the truth would have resulted in great pain and embarrassment for a number of perfectly innocent people. Beyond that, I could see no reason why the matter should be of public interest.

I had little doubt that an evasion or "no comment" would be taken as more than adequate confirmation by this particular writer, and no doubt whatsoever that there was no hope of successfully appealing to a sense of compassion and fair play. So I lied.

I did not just deny the allegation, but went to some trouble to construct a convincing argument as to what I suspected to be the case. Apparently, it worked, probably because others who were asked responded in much the same way I did. In any case, the story never appeared in print anywhere that I know of.

I have absolutely no regrets for what I did, and can say without hesitation that I would do the same thing again if similar circumstances arose. Quite simply, it seems to me that to the extent journalism insists upon the right to probe into matters that can destroy families and ruin careers, but which in no way involve a breach of public trust, it must also grant the right to those who become targets to defend themselves by the only means available.

Moreover, there will inevitably be a disputed area between journalists and public figures over what is, and what is not, a legitimate matter of public interest. In some cases, the answer may not be clear, even to the most unbiased observer, except in retrospect. And it hardly needs to be said that a *post hoc* decision that a personal matter should have remained private is of absolutely no benefit to those who have been hurt by its publication.

The other situation in which I believed, and still believe, that I had an obligation to lie occurred in April of 1980.

Following the collapse of the first of two attempts to negotiate an agreement with the Iranian government to secure the release of our hostages, because those nominally in positions of authority either could not or would not live up to their promises, the President began to look more seriously at a military rescue operation.

He had given orders for work to begin on such an option as soon as the hostages were seized. At that time, there seemed to be no feasible way to go about it with a decent chance of success. In the intervening months, as the Pentagon studied, planned, and trained, and as we learned more about the situation in the embassy compound through intelligence operations and the news media, the chances for a successful attempt began to increase.

Although I knew the work was being done, I knew nothing about its specifics, and indeed did not want to know, until March 22, 1980. In a meeting at Camp David to review our options following the disintegration of the first agreement, Secretary of Defense Brown and Joint Chiefs of Staff Chairman General David Jones presented a full briefing on their plans for a rescue operation.

It was impressive, both because of the work that had gone into it and the intelligence that we had managed to gather, and because the detailed consideration of such an option inevitably has a powerfully sobering effect on anyone with a say in whether or not it will be implemented.

Still, no one seemed to feel that this was the correct choice at the time. There were some questions raised about whether some aspects of what was necessarily a complex plan could not be simplified. More important in the decision not to go ahead then was the willingness, although reluctant, to give diplomacy one last chance. No one doubted that there would be American casualties, even in a successful operation. One Israeli soldier and three hostages had been killed at Entebbe, and the problem that faced our planners, and would face the strike force, were many times more difficult than anything the Israelis had confronted. There had also been messages from our intermediaries, and indirectly from Iranian officials, almost begging for a chance to put the negotiated agreement back on track.

Even though no one argued that day that we should choose the rescue option, I left the meeting feeling that we were heading down a road that would soon bring us to that choice unless the Iranians suddenly came to their senses. Despite my agreement with the decision to try the diplomatic approach again, I had to admit to myself that the odds seemed to be against the Iranians' implementing the agreement they had already reneged on once.

On the morning of April 11, shortly after that second diplomatic effort had indeed collapsed, the President called me into his office a few minutes before the regular Friday morning foreign-policy breakfast was to begin. During most of the administration, I had not attended these breakfasts on a regular basis. When the President felt that the agenda required my presence, he would let me know. Occasionally, I would ask to be included if I had a point I wanted to raise, or if I felt the need to listen to the discussion on a particular topic.

Once the hostage crisis began, however, I asked to attend on a regular basis, so that I could keep abreast of the latest thinking by the decision makers, as well as the often fast-breaking events. The President readily agreed. So I was somewhat surprised that morning when he said that he wanted to talk to me about whether I should attend the breakfast.

Then he explained that one of the topics, not included on the written agenda, was the rescue mission. I could tell, or thought I could, by his tone of voice and expression that this had now become a serious option for him.

Was this something I would rather not know about? the President asked. Would it make my job easier if down the road I could honestly claim to have had no knowledge of this option?

I replied that I had given some thought to the matter since the Camp David session. It seemed to me that if he decided to go ahead with the rescue option, we would need an aggressive effort to protect its secrecy. That might involve purposely misleading or even lying to the press. If it did, I was the person to do it. And if I did it, I wanted to have the information necessary to make my effort successful. Since I was also being asked about the Iran crisis almost every day, I said, there was the chance that I might inadvertently compromise the mission unless I knew exactly what activities were the most sensitive.

The President said he had expected that would be my response, and he agreed with it, but he had wanted to hear it from me.

Then he added with a hint of a smile, "If you have to lie to the press, I may have to fire you when this is all over, you know. I'm not sure I can have a press secretary who won't tell the truth to the press."

"That," I said, "would be doing me a real favor."

"And an even bigger one for the country," said the President with what I hoped was a smile, as he turned to walk to the Cabinet room, where his foreign policy team was waiting.

The briefing, on which I took no notes, was much the same as the earlier session at Camp David. Maps and charts were positioned on an easel and occasionally spread on the table for closer examination. The questions and suggestions from three weeks earlier had been taken into account, and the military planners had come up with a few new wrinkles on their own.

By the time it was over, I sensed that the men around the table, including the President, were leaning strongly toward ordering the plan to be implemented. The comments that followed confirmed my hunch. I added my endorsement, and emphasized again my feeling that we would need to give some thought to cover stories and an aggressive effort to protect the secrecy of the mission if the President decided to go ahead.

The only partial demurral came from Deputy Secretary of State Warren Christopher. Although he was inclined to recommend that the President order the mission, as he made clear later, he did not know how Secretary of State Vance (who was taking a brief and well-earned vacation) would react and did not feel that he should express a personal opinion.

The President said he was tentatively inclined to proceed

with the mission, but would defer a final decision until he had discussed it with Vance.

As we got up to leave the room, I found myself standing next to Harold Brown. "Mr. Secretary," I said, "the President is going to go with this thing, I can sense it. If we can bring our people out of there, it will do more good for this country than anything that has happened in twenty years."

"Yes," said Brown, "and if we fail, that will be the end of the Carter presidency."

"But we really don't have much choice, do we?"

The Secretary shook his head no as we walked out the door.

A moment later, Helen Thomas, of UPI, walked around the corner from the press room on the way to my office.

"Big meeting, huh?" she called down the short corridor. "You guys decide to nuke 'em?"

Brown and I both nodded yes, and I offered to let Helen and her colleagues know in plenty of time to be on the scene when the warheads struck.

If she only knew, I thought.

In fact, one of the problems we faced, once the President made his final decision four days later, was the number of press people in Tehran. As part of his objections, Cyrus Vance had warned that the Iranians might seize some of the several hundred Americans still in Tehran, thus leaving us with more hostages to worry about, even if the mission was a success. A fair number of this group were journalists.

I told the President that I saw no way for us to make the reporters come home, short of telling the news organizations what was about to happen, and that was clearly out of the question. Still, he felt an obligation to try. The President's first inclination was to order them home. I argued against this. There was no way to enforce the order, and I suspected that the attempt would so enrage the news executives that they would insist on keeping people there who might have been planning to come back anyway.

"Some of them are so ornery that they might just send an extra correspondent over to prove they can do it," I said.

In the end, we decided to use the increasingly volatile situation in Iran as an excuse to try to get journalists and other Americans to come home.

At a news conference on April 17, the President announced that he was prohibiting all financial transactions between Iranians and Americans and barring all imports from Iran. Then he stated that "to protect American citizens," he was banning all travel to Iran.

These steps, he said, would "not *now* be used to interfere with the right of the press to gather news.

"However," he continued, speaking slowly and precisely, "it is my responsibility and my obligation, given the situation in Iran, to call on American journalists and newsgathering organizations to minimize, as severely as possible, their presence and their activities in Iran."

As we had feared, the only effect was to provoke angry calls, particularly from the networks. After listening to Washington bureau chiefs and presidents of news divisions berate us for trying to repeal the First Amendment and stifle news coverage for political ends, I finally lost my temper with Sandy Socolow of CBS.

"Look Sandy," I said, "the President told you what he thinks you ought to do, and I have nothing to add to it. I warned him that you people would get on a high horse, but he wanted to do it anyway. I personally don't give a good goddamn what you people do. If I had my way, I'd ask the fucking Ayatollah to keep fifty reporters and give us our diplomats back. Then you people who have all the answers could figure out how to get them out."

As soon as I hung up the phone, I regretted having lost my temper. Not because I feared that I had hurt Socolow's feelings— he is not an overly sensitive fellow—but because I was worried that my angry response might have implied that something dramatic was about to happen. I had come that close to saying that he would have to accept the consequences for what happened if he ignored the President's warning, but had caught myself in time. I vowed to keep my temper in check, at least until this operation was complete.

The President's statement of April 17, in addition to being a futile attempt to get Americans out of Tehran, also fit into our cover story. By announcing additional sanctions, he implied that there would be a period of time during which we would wait and see if they would work before any other actions were taken. I, and others who knew what was actually afoot, strengthened this impression with background briefings.

We also suggested that if we were forced to consider any sort of military option, it would be something like a blockade or mining of harbors. This was the cover story we had devised for the military movements necessary to prepare for the rescue mission. On several occasions I speculated with reporters off the record about the relative merits of a blockade as opposed to mining.

We had, in fact, ruled out both of these options. They were unlikely to force the Iranians to yield, and once attempted would have to be followed up by an escalation of military force if no response was forthcoming. We would thus be starting down a road the end of which no one could see. We also believed that once any sort of military move was made, the Iranians as part of any general reaction might tighten security around the embassy, which we knew to be extremely lax, or disperse the hostages, thus denying us the rescue option.

The problems associated with the blockade were much the same as those associated with bombing power stations or other valuable targets in Iran—ideas that were being advanced by several columnists and commentators. I had suggested to the President earlier that what he ought to do was "bomb the hell out of every dam and power station in Iran. Let the Ayatollah shoot two hostages and call on the Russians for help, then turn the whole thing over to Agronsky and Company to handle."

His response is not printable.

By the week of April 20 it was becoming clear that our cover story was working too well. All the talk about mining and blockades was making some people nervous and everyone curious. That presented a problem. We did not want anyone, even on the White House staff, snooping around in an effort to find out what was going on. They just might stumble on something. In addition, once the staff begins to talk a great deal about anything, it is only a short time before the press gets interested, too.

But this also presented us with an opportunity to reinforce our cover story. On Tuesday, April 22, little more than forty-eight hours before the Delta Team would enter Iranian air space, Hamilton called a staff meeting to address the concerns that were buzzing about the staff. He assured them all that we had no plans, at the moment, for mining or blockading. When asked about a rescue mission, he lied.

As soon as I heard what had taken place, I began to prepare for a press call. It came less than ninety minutes after the meeting ended. Jack Nelson, bureau chief of the *Los Angeles Times*, wanted to talk to me about something he had heard from a "pretty interesting staff meeting you people had this morning." I said I had not been there but would check with Hamilton.

I then called Hamilton to tell him what I was about to do. I hated to do it to Nelson, who was one of the more decent journalists that I had gotten to know since coming to Washington, and one who would become a good friend once the administration was over. But I did not feel that I had any choice. I knew what he wanted to talk about. It was an opportunity to reinforce the web of deception we had constructed to protect the rescue mission.

When I called Nelson back, he said he had heard that some staffers had expressed concern that we were about to take some action that might "involve us in a war." I confirmed this report and repeated Hamilton's assurances that we were planning no military action whatsoever, and certainly nothing like a rescue mission.

Later that day, Nelson came by my office to continue our discussion. Toward the end of that conversation, he asked, "You people really aren't thinking about doing anything drastic like launching a rescue mission, are you?"

This was the moment of truth, or, more accurately, of deception. Up to this point, I had only repeated false statements made by others, an admittedly fine distinction, but a distinction nevertheless. Now I was faced with a direct question. With a swallow that I hoped was not noticeable, I began to recite all the reasons why a rescue operation would not make any sense. They were familiar because they were exactly the ones that it had taken four months to figure out how to overcome.

"If and when we are forced to move militarily, I suspect it will be something like a blockade," I said, "but that decision is a step or two down the road."

I made a mental note to be sure to call Jack and apologize once the operation was completed, hoping he would understand.

The result was a story in the *Los Angeles Times* reporting Hamilton's assurances to the staff that no military action was in the offing, and that a rescue operation was still considered to be impractical.

When I read it the next day, I remember hoping that some Iranian student at Berkeley had enough loyalty to the Ayatollah to phone it in to Tehran.

Two days later the hostage rescue attempt ended in disaster. Nelson, to his credit, seemed to understand what I had done, even though he could not explicitly condone it. Most other reporters reacted in similar fashion when the story of my deception came out. A few even stopped by to say privately that they would have done the same thing in my position. A few others were quoted, anonymously, as saying that I had destroyed my credibility and ought to resign.

The issue quickly faded as we dealt with the spectacle of Iranian leaders boasting over the bodies of American servicemen, the tortured but eventually successful efforts to secure their return, and the ceremonies honoring their courage and dedication to duty.

There were a few attempts to exploit the situation for political purposes: stories were planted with reporters that the mission had been discovered by the Soviets and a call from Brezhnev had brought about the cancellation, and that the military commanders had wanted to go ahead after the loss of three helicopters but the President had lost his nerve and ordered them to turn back. These attempts at disinformation were largely unsuccessful. Later, as we shall see, those responsible for these efforts were able to find journalists whose indifference or incompetence made them useful political tools.

In October of 1983, as this book was being finished, controversy flared again between the White House and the press over the relative rights and responsibilities of the two institutions. The occasion was the American invasion of Grenada, and there were several reasonably separate issues involved.

The first was the same one that I had dealt with three and a half years prior: the right of government to lie. On the afternoon before American forces landed in Grenada, CBS White House correspondent Bill Plante learned from a reliable source that an invasion would take place at sunrise the next morning. He checked with the White House Press Office and got a flat denial.

"Preposterous," said spokesman Larry Speakes. Other reporters got the same response from other government officials.

The decision by the Reagan administration to deceive journalists rather than risk the possibility that the invasion plans would be disclosed seemed to me to be eminently defensible.

When I asked Plante later what he would have done if the White House had confirmed the invasion plans, his response was "I don't know; we would have tried to find some way to use what we knew without endangering the operation."

That in itself would seem to confirm the wisdom of the White House judgment. You cannot expect government to leave such questions in the hands of the fourth estate. The consequences of an error are too severe.

Moreover, given the extent of eavesdropping capabilities in Washington, it would be an unacceptable risk to have Mr. Plante and others at CBS chatting at some length over open telephone lines about how they would use the information. By the time their decision was made it most likely would be moot.

Some journalists were willing to agree privately that this situation was one of those in which there was no other choice but to lie. Most, however, were unwilling to endorse publicly the idea that lying could be condoned under any circumstances, feeling that government does enough lying as it is without any encouragement from them.

They make the very valid point that once you step away from the categorical, there is no easily discernible place to draw the line.

Still the essential dilemma remains. What about those situations where an evasion simply will not work, where a "no comment" is almost certain to be taken as a confirmation? If, at the same time, the information to be protected is of sufficient importance, if lives are at stake for example, a lie becomes in my estimation the lesser evil of the choices available. It is ludicrous to argue that soldiers may be sent off to fight and die, but a spokesman may not, under any circumstances, be asked to lie to make sure that the casualties are fewer and not in vain.

Churchill made the point with his usual flair in 1943. "In wartime," he said, "truth is so precious that she should be attended by a bodyguard of lies."

Unfortunately, once one steps onto the slippery slope of relativism, firm footing cannot be established, even on the basis of "wartime" or "lives at stake." There are other dilemmas that can and do arise, where calculated deception might be appropriate.

Although I never faced it personally, the protection of an important intelligence source or method, even in peacetime, might be one.

And what about the protection of an important diplomatic initiative? I almost faced such a situation at Camp David when reports of bad blood between Sadat and Begin arose and when there were leaks about Sadat's threat to break off the talks. As described earlier in this book, I was able to deal with those problems without telling a bald-faced lie, but that was mostly a matter of luck.

In the midst of the Grenada controversy, a columnist revealed that the premature publication by Jack Anderson of a story about Henry Kissinger's secret diplomatic initiatives had damaged, although not fatally, the movement toward normalization of relations with China. That initiative became arguably the most significant strategic event since the Second World War. Would lying have been appropriate in an effort to keep it on track?

In the early months of the Carter administration the *Washington Post* published accounts of secret payments through the CIA to King Hussein of Jordan. The story appeared on the day that Secretary of State Vance arrived in Amman to discuss a Middle East peace initiative with Hussein. Needless to say, the result was a less than positive environment for the talks.

In that case, we had chosen to be candid with the *Post* and appeal to their sense of responsibility. From our point of view the effort was a failure. Although we had not asked them not to publish the story, feeling that such a request would be futile, we had requested a delay. When it came out at the most unfortunate of all possible times, we felt the *Post* was guilty of bad faith. The *Post* maintained that the timing was a result of a misunderstanding.

In any case, the question remains. In our judgment the *Post* had enough information to go with the story whatever we said. But what if we had concluded that it was possible to kill the story with a lie, would we have been justified in doing so?

To take another step down the slope, what degree of deception would be acceptable from a Justice Department official trying to protect the rights of an innocent person whose name had cropped up in an investigation?

Or what about a spokesman at Treasury attempting to avoid the premature disclosure of information on a financial decision that could lead to severe damage to innocent parties and great profits for those in a position to take advantage of the leak?

The problem becomes, as noted above, where precisely to draw the line. There is no convenient place. About the best one can do is to argue that it must be drawn very tightly, for practical as well as moral considerations. Distinctions may be difficult at the margins, but we can all tell the difference between mountains and molehills. If government does have the right to lie in certain situations, that right is as precious as the truth it attends. It must not be squandered on matters of less than overriding importance.

Which brings us to another issue in the Grenada controversy. Many correspondents said that the exchange between Speakes and CBS was not the cause but the catalyst for their outrage. They charged that the administration had repeatedly lied to them on matters that were in no way vital to national security or the protection of lives. They listed examples that ranged from the dates of resignations to travel plans to attempts to square the facts with some off-the-cuff presidential remark.

They also pointed to a history of efforts to curtail the flow of information, from the screening of calls to White House officials from reporters by the communications and press offices to proposals for the review of anything written by thousands of government officials after they leave office. (At this writing, Congress has wisely blocked this last absurdity, but the administration has vowed not to give up.)

That attitude was not unanimous, but it was clearly shared by a large number of White House correspondents. And that is a dangerous set of circumstances for the administration and potentially for the nation. The danger for the administration is that it will find itself lacking credibility across the board, that no explanation will be accepted at face value and every action will be subject to the most unflattering interpretation.

For the nation, the danger lies in the fact that an administration that is generally believed to be dishonest will not command the respect necessary to protect legitimate secrets. There are many cases in which truths less vital than the timing and objective of military operations are protected by successful appeals to reporters not to publish. The full and exact reasons for such requests cannot always be disclosed, because they too may be quite sensitive. Needless to say, such appeals—which amount to a request to "trust me"—can only be effective in a climate of mutual trust.

To the extent that this climate was placed in jeopardy following the Grenada controversy, the problem was not primarily a conflict over government's right to lie about issues of ultimate importance, but a perceived pattern of deception solely for the sake of convenience—of lies designed to protect and promote nothing more precious than someone's political backside.

Even during the Grenada operation, there were lies from the government that were difficult to justify by any reasonable standard. Claims that coverage was curtailed, after the invasion had begun, because of concern for the safety of reporters were poppycock. Even experienced spokesmen had a hard time making that argument with a straight face.

Similarly, attempts to blame the decision to restrict coverage on "military commanders" were deceptive and cowardly and dangerous. There is no doubt that many uniformed military officers hold the press in less than great esteem or that the restricted coverage was completely in line with their preferences. But that is not the point. Such decisions are always subject to White House review. And they were repeatedly brought to the attention of White House officials. If the preferences of the military commanders were honored, it was because the President and his men agreed with them.

This refusal to accept responsibility for one's own actions was dangerous in this case because it served to exacerbate tensions between the military and the fourth estate, to heighten mutual distrust on both sides. These tensions are already high enough and that problem is going to be with us for the indefinite future. Already it works against responsible and accurate reporting of national security issues. It also promotes an unreasoning distrust of all things military in our society. There is, in my view, no excuse for an administration's hiding behind the armed forces simply to avoid facing ticklish questions.

A related issue has to do with how much the White House press secretary should be told in situations such as this. It very quickly became clear in this particular case that the press secretary and the press office had been kept in the dark until the invasion was under way. Mr. Speakes and his people were not intentionally lying themselves when they denied the reports from Plante and other newsmen; they were merely passing on what they had been told by members of the National Security Council staff.

This quickly became a bone of contention within the White House. Mr. Speakes and his people were none too happy about the way they had been treated. One deputy resigned as a result. However, more senior White House officials declared themselves well pleased with the procedure and stated that they would handle things the same way if similar situations arose in the future.

Mr. Speakes made it clear that if a lie was required and he was to be sent out to tell it, he wanted to know what was at stake. And he was exactly right. Keeping the press secretary in the dark can create serious problems.

First, it inevitably erodes the press secretary's effectiveness. It costs him in prestige and status, factors that may mean more than they should in Washington, but still cannot be ignored. The press secretary's job is tough enough as it is; he deserves every break his colleagues can give him. Putting the guy whose business is information in a position that makes him appear to be uninformed, out of touch, and not trusted makes no sense over the long haul.

Beyond that, if a secret is worth lying about to protect, it makes sense to come up with the most effective lie possible. Most sensitive operations are accompanied by a cover story, designed to provide an innocent explanation for bits and pieces that might leak out. Since the first group of people that such a story must convince is the press, having the press secretary involved in designing the story is not a bad idea. He more than anyone else is likely to know what will be convincing and what will not.

Furthermore, the use of the story, if it ever becomes necessary, is likely to be more effective if the person who puts it out knows exactly what he is trying to do. Dealing with the press, particularly in ticklish situations, is very much an art. You cannot treat the press secretary like a robot and then expect him to perform like an artist.

Another danger in keeping the press secretary uninformed comes from the way in which a press office operates. When a new question arises or an issue looks like it is going to get hot, the press office begins to function very much like a news organization. Deputy and assistant and deputy assistant press secretaries immediately get to work calling all over the government to try to find out what is really going on and where it may lead.

As information is gathered, it is often passed on to the reporter who has made the query in bits and pieces as part of a continuing exchange of information and ideas. Needless to say, if there is something highly sensitive that has to be protected, the press secretary needs to know about it. Otherwise, this process could stumble into and lead to the uncovering of information that should be kept secret.

In matters large and small, keeping the press secretary in the dark is risky business. If he cannot be trusted with sensitive information, he should be replaced. Failing that, he ought to be given the information he needs to do his job effectively.

Having said all that, however, I suspect that the most important lesson from this episode is to be found in the fact that the press was a clear loser in its fight with the administration over Grenada. It lost in the court in which such matters will eventually be decided—the court of public opinion. In the immediate aftermath of Grenada it was sometimes difficult to tell which the American people enjoyed more, seeing the President kick hell out of the Cubans or the press.

And the reasons the fourth estate lost were to a large extent its own fault.

The strength of the public reaction in favor of the administration's policy of denying access to the press was a shock to many Washington journalists. The more thoughtful were concerned as well as surprised.

It is true that the press is particularly vulnerable among our major institutions because it is so often the bearer of sad tidings, the forum for criticism of ideas, individuals, and institutions that Americans hold dear. It is also true, as journalists are fond of pointing out, that their job is not to win popularity contests. But the vocal and sometimes vicious public reaction against the press in the wake of Grenada was more than just some sort of "shoot the messenger" syndrome.

In part it sprang from the way the fourth estate handled the terrorist bombing of our marine headquarters in Beirut, which occurred just prior to the Grenada operation. The behavior of some news organizations was not the sort that would inspire public confidence in their judgment or self-restraint.

There was, for example, the repugnant spectacle of CBS camped ghoulishly at the home of parents awaiting word on the fate of their marine son in Beirut. And they hit the jackpot. The boy was dead. So they got to film the arrival of the casualty officer and the chaplain bringing the tragic news to the parents.

The tragic scene, for which every standard of good taste and decency demanded privacy, was then offered up to satisfy the voyeurism of the worst segments of the American television audience and the demands for the higher ratings that are believed, with some justification, to come with sensationalism.

Nor was this sort of gross insensitivity confined to television. A few days after the Beirut bombing, readers of the *Washington Post* were treated to the incredibly insensitive comments of a *Newsweek* executive describing at some length what a wonderful thing the tragedy was for his magazine:

"We are exhilarated by this. It's the sort of thing *Newsweek* does best—react to a big story in a big way. We'll be pulling out all the stops. . . . one hell of a story . . . pursuing a variety of angles . . . expect a lot of competition, it's the biggest story of the year."

If the tasteless coverage of the Beirut tragedy was a factor in the public's reaction to Grenada, it was by no means the whole of it. The attitudes reflected did not develop over a few days or weeks.

If the government has in this and other instances been guilty of excess in the exercise of what I believe to be its legitimate right to mislead and even deceive on matters of vital import, the fourth estate has also been guilty of excess in its cavalier insistence on the right to do as it pleases with little regard for good judgment, good taste, or the consequences of its actions—and the American people know it.

One consequence of the information explosion has been that more and more Americans have had the opportunity to see news coverage of incidents they knew something about. And they have come away disillusioned, and sometimes angry, because of the wide gap that too often existed between what they knew to be the case and what was reported.

And if they were foolish enough to try to set the record straight by appealing for a correction, they also ran head on into that determination never to admit a mistake, much less do anything about it.

The public's reaction to Grenada ought to be a danger signal for journalism. The question that will not be answered until after this book goes to press is how the fourth estate will react. The greatest danger is that the reaction will be defensive, a renewed determination to pretend that nothing is wrong except the shortsightedness and lack of sophistication of the American public. What the reaction ought to be, at least in the opinion of this writer, is the subject of the chapter on recommendations near the end of this book.

FEAR AND LOATHING
IN NEW YORK⎯⎯⎯⎯⎯⎯

A s spring of 1980 turned into summer and the Democratic
convention approached, the President continued to pile up
delegates, but our relations with the press oscillated between bad and abysmal. According to Robinson and Sheehan,
Carter's press index from April through July was −51, −35,
−14, and −29 with CBS. In stark contrast, Kennedy's CBS rating for the same four-month period was decidedly positive.

From the perspective of the press office, the odds for our final
confrontation with Kennedy did not look encouraging. Nor was I
terribly happy about the site. I had first learned of the location for
the convention almost a year earlier. In the fall of 1979, during
our regular morning meeting, the President asked out of the blue
what I thought about holding the 1980 Democratic convention in
New York. My first reaction was less than enthusiastic. I had
hoped that we could find some way to hold the convention in the
South. But the prohibition against meeting in any state that had
not ratified the Equal Rights Amendment—a typical cut-off-your-
nose-to-spite-your-face party rule—had made that impossible.

Still, New York did not excite me. I was even then convinced
that we would be facing a challenge by Kennedy. If the first President from the Deep South in a century and a quarter was to
mount a last-ditch fight for his political life, surely there was a
better place than New York.

There was also the matter of then Governor Hugh Carey and
New York City Mayor Ed Koch. No more slippery pair of political ingrates had ever sidled into the Oval Office, hat in one hand,

shiv in the other. To me, they epitomized what was wrong with American politics and the Democratic party: they were self-serving, unscrupulous, and congenitally unable to accept the responsibility for their own problems.

Carter had saved Koch and his city from financial disaster, a not altogether popular move in the rest of the country. Yet Koch never missed an opportunity to spit in the hand that fed him. There was something about the man that reminded me of our old nemesis Lester Maddox. It was not just the bald head and glasses, although the physical resemblance was something striking. The political style also brought back old and not very pleasant memories. The playing of ethnic and racial groups against one another. The practiced buffoonery and outrageous comment. Even the incessant whining about how the federal government was responsible for all his problems. All made me think of old Lester every time I saw the distinguished mayor of New York.

To be fair, however, the two men are not the same. If I had to loan one five dollars or ask one to watch my house while I was on vacation, I'd go with Lester every time.

For his part, Carey had directed most of his efforts toward making sure that the state government accepted as little of the responsibility as possible for the problems of the city, while deriving the maximum political benefit.

The fact that Carey and Koch seemed to despise each other, and spent a good part of their time at the White House talking about what a rascal the other was, only confirmed to me the old maxim that it takes one to know one.

The President listened to my tirade with a bemused smile. He seldom gave vent to his feelings about others in front of his staff. He seemed to feel that such outbursts set a bad example. The closest he came to violating that rule was after a lengthy conversation with the mayor. The President sat in silence for a moment, then said, to no one in particular, "I don't believe I ever met a man so completely wrapped up in himself."

When I had finished, he explained that it was because of Carey and Koch that he was leaning toward the Big Apple. Both had promised their unqualified support for his renomination in return for holding the convention in New York.

That changed my mind in a hurry. In the first place, it made sense to site the convention in a place where a Democratic mayor and governor were supporting the President. Beyond that, they could be extremely helpful to us in a fight with Kennedy.

It did cross my mind that getting a commitment from those two and getting it fulfilled had often proven to be two different things entirely. Nevertheless, it seemed like the best deal we were likely to get.

As it turned out, both of them ended up supporting the President, but only after a fashion. And their support did considerably more damage than if they had been in outright opposition. Carey played footsie with Kennedy privately and occasionally in public throughout the nomination fight, never giving his endorsement until it was over. Koch even agreed to Reagan's request for a very public breakfast shortly before the general election. It was a signal to millions of New Yorkers that their mayor could work with the man if he became president, something Koch had to know when he agreed to do it.

As a result, my reaction to the mayor's anguished cries, as support for his city was slashed by his 1980 breakfast buddy, has been somewhat ambivalent to say the least. Nor did it seem to me to be a great tragedy when Koch lost the 1982 Democratic primary for governor, in part due to his reputation as Ronald Reagan's favorite Democratic mayor.

But Koch and Carey were only a small part of the problems we faced at the 1980 convention. It was a long-running, nationally televised disaster from beginning to end. It provided a platform and an opportunity for Kennedy to keep his political ambitions alive and to inflict as much damage as possible on the President, who had refused to turn the White House over to him.

It had been clear to most observers since the end of April that it was all but mathematically impossible for Kennedy to win the nomination. But this did not prompt the senator to withdraw gracefully and begin the process of healing wounds before we had to face Ronald Reagan in the fall.

Instead, he seemed to be bent upon finding any excuse to keep his challenge in motion, even if it could not be kept alive. What he came up with was the idea of changing the party rules so that the results of the primaries and caucuses could be disregarded at the convention.

Under the banner of an "open convention," he crusaded for a new rule that would allow delegates to disregard the wishes of those who had elected them and vote for anyone they chose. We decided to fight on the issue, primarily because caving in would have given an appearance of weakness. But I cannot deny that we were also in a fighting mood. We had made every effort to offer Kennedy an honorable way out and we had borne in silence a series of indignities as we tried to work with his staff to schedule a meeting between the two men once the primaries were over. Now, we were genuinely and totally upset by his determination to stay in the spotlight, no matter what the cost to the party or the "issues" that were supposedly so close to his heart.

We tried to make the argument that there was something pre-adolescent about a loser pitching a temper tantrum and screaming for a change in the rules after the game was over. On one occasion we even asked journalists to consider for a moment what their reaction would have been if Carter had tried such a thing.

But of course Carter was that sly, manipulative politician who was only looking out after his own hide. Teddy was something else, a dedicated, compassionate statesman of unquestioned integrity whose only concern was the welfare of his party and the country. If he occasionally behaved in ways that would have gotten other politicians ridden out of town on a rail, thoughtful observers would note that it was in a good cause. Only an insensitive jerk would make an issue of it.

The truth of the matter was that most of the delegates were totally unknown to the voters who had elected them. They were at the convention for one reason, their pledge to support a particular candidate for the presidential nomination. The idea that they had been elected to exercise their independent judgment on this question in some Burkean sense was absurd on its face. But absurdity seldom is allowed to get in the way of a good story.

Instead of getting ready for a successful convention and preparing for the general election, we were forced to divert time and resources to the "open convention" fight. Although the issue was never really in doubt, we were running scared. That suited the press and the Kennedy camp just fine. About every three days, the Kennedy camp would produce a new delegate total showing that their strength was growing. They were all bogus, but the press ran with them anyway. Time after time we urged journalists to ask for the names of the delegates who were supposedly jumping ship. A few did. As we had expected, few names were given.

It soon became obvious to even the most trusting that the Kennedy people were misrepresenting the facts, but no journalist called them on it. Still, the "open convention gains momentum" stories continued to crop up. The whole thing was particularly galling to me since I had insisted that we be scrupulously correct in our delegate count claims. My argument was that if we were caught in an error, even an honest one, our credibility would be shot. And I have no doubt that it would have been.

There is no denying that some of the problems we experienced leading up to and during the convention were our own fault. Our mistakes stemmed from two misconceptions.

We underestimated the antipathy of the Democratic interest groups and the party's left wing. Surely, we thought, they can see what a disaster a Reagan presidency would be for the people they are supposed to represent. They have a stake in not turning this thing into a debacle. And they must have learned from the 1972 convention how much a plank in a losing platform is worth.

We also misread Kennedy's attitude. Despite considerable evidence to the contrary, we had always figured that when it was all over he would do his best on behalf of the Democratic ticket. He had, it was true, refused to pledge himself to support the nominee of the party during the primaries. At the time it rankled us, because Carter had made it clear from the beginning that as a loyal Democrat he would support Kennedy if he won the nomination.

Still, we figured that his position during the primaries was mostly an effort to keep his supporters fired up and maintain a consistent theme. It is hard to say in one breath that a man is destroying the country, leading us into war, and snatching food from the mouths of hungry children, and promise to support him in the next. Whatever his differences with Carter, those with Reagan were so much greater that he surely would rally to the banner in the fall. Or so we thought.

I am convinced, in retrospect, that we neglected to take into account one of the most obvious facets of Kennedy's character, an almost childlike self-centeredness. His whole career had been marked by the indulgence of personal whims, with little apparent regard for the long-term consequences—for himself or others.

It should have been obvious to us that a Carter victory in 1980 was not in Kennedy's best interests. By 1984, Mondale would surely be the odds-on favorite for the nomination. There was also the historical tendency of the country not to give the same party more than eight years in the White House. If Carter won in 1980 and a Republican won in 1984, it might well be 1992 before Edward M. Kennedy had another good shot at the presidency.

We also thought that Kennedy would not risk the criticism that would certainly come his way if his petulance helped to elect Reagan in 1980. Hadn't Carter been grilled over and over again about the strength of his support of McGovern in 1972? (He had announced that he would support the Democratic ticket, invited McGovern to Georgia, and welcomed him when he came, but had not stumped the state for him, which would have been a rather futile effort at best.)

Surely, an attempt to sabotage Carter's reelection efforts would become an issue in its own right and damage the senator's prospects for the future. On this point, we simply forget that Teddy Kennedy is not held to the same standards as other politicians.

Indeed the sabotaging of Carter was at its most visible at the convention and in the weeks just prior, but it never became an item of discussion in the media.

Part of the Kennedy strategy was quite simply to hold the Democratic party hostage. His first move was to file a deluge of minority reports on the platform, most of them totally frivolous. Under the party rules, he could demand debate and a vote on each one. In short, he could wreck the convention by making sure prime time was filled with wrangling and divisive debate, and that the President's acceptance speech was delayed until the wee hours of the morning.

His other tactic was to play footsie with independent presidential candidate John Anderson, savior of the nation, darling of the press, and at the time a serious threat to the Democratic ticket, whoever was on it. Two weeks before the convention opened, Anderson and Kennedy met at Kennedy's office for a well-publicized orgy of mutual admiration.

Anderson did his part by hinting that he might not be a candidate in the general election if Kennedy was the Democratic nominee (a comment that would have destroyed the market in Brie futures had it been taken seriously). Kennedy mugged for the cameras and heaped praise on the "responsible solutions" that Anderson was advocating. Fortunately for them both, the reporters in attendance were too dazzled by this display of intellectual prostitution to ask the senator to name one.

The message of the Anderson flirtation was clear. If I don't get my way, I'll spend the fall talking about what a wonderful fellow John Anderson is.

The press, as one might expect, was beside itself. Here were two of their favorite politicians snuggling up to each other in public. The truth was that the only news in it was the length to which both men were prepared to go to advance their personal ambitions. But it would have been crass of any journalist to raise such a discomfiting thought on such an inspiring occasion.

Our final mistake, which flowed logically from the others, was the way we approached the Kennedy challenge at the convention. Thinking that he might, despite all evidence to the contrary, be only looking for an honorable way out, enough satisfaction from the platform and the convention proceedings to allow him to declare his campaign effort not in vain, we were determined to be doggedly conciliatory.

The result of these fundamental misapprehensions was that we got taken to the cleaners. Each time we made a concession on the platform or the convention schedule, Teddy's people had another demand ready to toss on the table.

It was always something that was "particularly important to the senator," something he just had to have "if he was going to be able, in good conscience, to support the ticket enthusiastically."

In this case, the press correctly sensed the atmosphere. We had the nomination locked up, but we were nevertheless on the defensive. There was a sour odor of frustration and recrimination in the air that sent the nostrils of journalists flaring the moment they hit town.

Time and again we accepted platform provisions that we did not like, because we thought they were wrong-headed and because we knew they would be political liabilities in the campaign against the GOP. It was not just because of the value we placed on Kennedy's support in the fall, but because we were trying to keep the convention from turning into a divisive spectacle.

Looking back, I cannot help but wish we had told him and his people to kiss off. We might well have lost the election anyway. The senator might well have followed through on his threats to snuggle up to John Anderson, thus drawing more liberal votes away from the ticket. We certainly would have lost a number of floor fights over platform planks. But we probably would have been better off repudiating the document anyway. It was, in some ways, as fiscally irresponsible on the left as Reagan's proposals were on the right. Whatever the political consequences, we would have delivered a message to Teddy that he very much needed to hear. The Democratic party might well have been better off in the long run. And we would have felt a great deal better about ourselves.

The night of Carter's acceptance speech summed up the whole miserable affair. Kennedy had wowed the crowd with what was supposed to be a withdrawal speech two nights before. In the process he had stampeded the delegates into approving an economic package that was one part dreams and two parts foolishness. We had been forced to swallow a plank calling for a $12 billion jobs program and another that gave too little attention to the problems of inflation. Only by skillful horse trading had we avoided a wage-and-price-controls provision—a plank that the President would have been forced to repudiate publicly.

Carter could not match the senator's rhetorical skills. Nor was he about to make the kind of substantive commitments that Senator Kennedy and his hard-core delegates wanted to hear.

We had urged our people to respond positively to Kennedy's speech—that old "They'll come around if we're nice to them" fallacy again. Most of the Kennedy delegates sat on their hands during the Carter speech.

Nevertheless, it was a more than adequate performance. It was not Carter's best, but it was good enough for our purposes. The start was a bit shaky, primarily because of problems with the TelePrompTer, but as the President moved along he warmed to his task. He hit squarely and with conviction, again and again, on the themes and issues we had chosen for the fall campaign. Coupled with the Vice-President's purposely more partisan presentation earlier that evening, it conveyed the message we would need to drive home to beat Ronald Reagan.

As it ended, I breathed a sigh of relief. At least the thing was over. There was little doubt in my mind that we would get the traditional postconvention boost in the polls, despite the bitter taste the proceedings had left in my mouth. In a few days, the polls would substantiate that assumption. Carter had closed the margin from a −16 just before the convention to a dead heat the week after.

But it was not over. There were still the postspeech formalities to get through, and they would become the enduring symbol of the 1980 convention.

The Kennedy people had, on several occasions, expressed doubt about whether he would appear on the platform with the President after the acceptance speech to offer the traditional congratulations and pledge of support. Failure to do so would have been a clear declaration of nonsupport for the ticket, something we were not anxious to see as the final act of the convention. But that had been settled the day before, or so we thought.

Once the senator graciously agreed to show up, there was some discussion about the logistics of getting him to the podium. He insisted that he watch the speech in his hotel suite. The VIP suite at Madison Square Garden did not suit his taste. We were wary enough by then to fear that he would emerge from his hotel before the speech was over, tempting the networks to cut away from the President, particularly if he stopped to make a few comments to the live cameras stationed at his hotel door.

As a result, it was agreed that he would leave his hotel as soon as the speech was over. That meant it would be a few minutes before he could make it to the platform, but the time could easily be filled.

As it turned out, the trip from the Waldorf-Astoria to the Garden took about twice as long as we had anticipated. The senator could have made better time on a skateboard. The situation on the podium began to get awkward.

Bob Strauss, a master at making the best of such situations, had long since run through his list of dignitaries to be called up to shake hands with Carter and Mondale. He was winging it in a way that only he knows how to do, but it was obvious that even

Strauss could not reel off the names of politicos from the top of his head indefinitely.

When Kennedy finally arrived, things moved rapidly from awkward to painful. As he watched President Carter's acceptance speech, the senator and his aides had come up with one final indignity to inflict on the nominee of their party. Laughing and joking about what a spectacle it would be on prime-time television, they began to act out the contortions that the senator would go through to deny the President the traditional raised handclasp, the symbol of party unity.

After the election, some of those aides took great glee in describing at length how they had choreographed the senator's final performance of the 1980 convention.

It worked like a charm. From the floor where I was sitting, the awkwardness it caused was not particularly noticeable, but for those watching on television, it was clear that something was amiss.

The President, never suspecting that he was being used in one final display of adolescent peevishness, kept looking around, reaching for the senator's arm with his eyes if not with his hand. Each time Teddy would dance away. Twice Kennedy came up to the podium where the President and Vice-President stood. Twice he turned aside, studiously avoiding the signal that their bitter fight had ended and the party would face the Republicans united. It looked awful, and it was.

I did not realize what a disaster it had been until I entered the press area after the convention had been gaveled to a close. Reporters were talking about nothing else. Gone was the impact of the President and Vice-President's carefully coordinated presentation of our fall campaign themes. Gone too was any chance that a positive and upbeat conclusion would erase some of the negativism generated by the depressing days just prior.

To make sure that none of the reporters had missed the snub, Kennedy's staff had tipped off a few of their spear carriers in the press, who had done their job of passing the word to their colleagues. Not that any reasonably astute political observer who had seen the spectacle on television needed to be told that it was not an accident.

My first reaction was outrage, not at Kennedy, but at the

press. This was the big night of the convention. Despite it all, we had won, dammit, and here they were, all aflutter over a handshake. What they knew and I did not, of course, was that it had all been preplanned. And many of them had also seen the consequences on television.

As it turned out, the next day's stories did not feature the handshake fiasco as prominently as I had expected. It had happened too late in the evening for most editions of morning papers. But those that did mention it predictably focused on Carter's discomfort and awkwardness, rather than Kennedy's childishness. My arguments that most decent people will appear ill at ease when unexpectedly confronted with loutish behavior were singularly unpersuasive.

The effect was not so much the coverage that the incident received but the mood it created among the press. The President's acceptance speech had been surprisingly successful in its immediate impact on the public, as the polls soon demonstrated. (Just prior to the convention, Gallup showed Reagan holding a 45-29 lead with Anderson at 14. Postconvention, Gallup found the race a dead heat with Reagan at 38, Carter at 39, and Anderson at 13.) But it had left a bitter taste and an air of negativism among all those who attended, including and most importantly those who would be reporting on the campaign for the next two months.

DISINFORMATION _____

While we were struggling to deal with the quite visible attacks from the left wing of our own party, the Republicans were not just sitting back to enjoy the spectacle. They had plans of their own, less public, but every bit as dangerous as and considerably more vicious than those concocted by the Kennedy faction.

As the Democratic convention began, so did a campaign of disinformation using forged intelligence documents and operatives inside the government to deceive reporters and embarrass the administration.

It is not possible to determine exactly who was responsible for each of the several attempts to spread damaging falsehoods and half-truths. Some reporters still refuse to divulge the names of their sources, even though they now admit the information they received from them was false. Others say they received the documents and tips anonymously, never knowing exactly where they originated.

It is possible, however, to identify at least one group of government officials that was involved in the spreading of disinformation in a manner that had all the hallmarks of a calculated and well-orchestrated campaign. In January of 1980, a group of ultra-conservative Senate staffers met for lunch at the Madison Hotel in downtown Washington. They formed a group that met every other Friday for lunch. It came to be known as the Madison Group, and its purpose—in the words of columnist William Safire—was to "embarrass, bedevil, and defeat" the Carter administration. Part of what they were up to is standard procedure for Washington politics, the pooling of information and the leaking of potentially embarrassing tidbits to the press.

But the Madison Group was not content with such routine tactics. Their behavior went well beyond standard rumor mongering. Making use of high-level security clearances, which they held because of their staff positions on sensitive congressional committees, they planned and executed a campaign featuring concocted stories based upon nonexistent or totally misrepresented classified documents and information.

Once the presidential campaign began in earnest, they established a liaison with the Reagan campaign in the person of Charles Kupperman. His contact in the Reagan camp was the candidate's principal foreign-policy adviser, Richard Allen, who later became President Reagan's adviser for national security affairs. Neither Mr. Allen nor the members of the group are willing to discuss how closely the activities of the Madison Group were coordinated with the campaign or how much campaign officials knew about specific projects.

What is clear is that the group was not without considerable resources. Not only did their intelligence clearances provide access to extremely sensitive information, but they could also call upon ideological soul mates within the executive branch to assist in their projects.

What is also clear is that individuals closely connected with the Reagan campaign were involved in disinformation, often of the same type as and involving subjects similar to that put out by the Madison Group.

In most cases, journalists were too smart to be taken in, but not always. In a few instances, they seemed to be disinclined to risk ruining a good story by checking it too closely.

The most spectacular success was a totally fabricated story that Jack Anderson swallowed whole. It resulted in a series of columns by Anderson that appeared in hundreds of newspapers across the country, just as the Democratic convention was ending.

The information that Anderson claimed to have was a bombshell: proof that President Carter was planning an invasion of Iran just before the election, an invasion that moreover was opposed by his military advisers, who, according to Anderson's columns, believed that the President was simply trying to provoke an international crisis to ensure his reelection.

In early August of 1980, Anderson says, he was presented

with documents detailing a plan for a mid-October invasion of Iran. The documents also showed that President Carter had tentatively approved the invasion date. And, according to Anderson, both the decision and the date were confirmed by an anonymous source who worked on the National Security Council staff in the Carter White House.

What was more, Anderson claimed that his unnamed NSC source had also revealed the reason for the invasion: the President had ordered it "to save himself from . . . defeat in November." From August 18 through August 22, Anderson wrote and distributed no less than six consecutive columns, pounding away at this allegation.

Had it been true, Anderson would have had the scoop of the century. The President's alleged actions were not only insane, but probably impeachable offenses. Anderson was certainly correct on one point: any idea of a "full-scale invasion of Iran" would have been unanimously opposed by civilian as well as military advisers. Had the President issued such orders, he might well have faced mass resignations at the Pentagon and at the White House.

But the allegation was totally false, a fabrication from start to finish, and a particularly vicious one at that. The President of the United States was depicted as a man who would send thousands of Americans to die in combat and risk war with the Soviet Union simply because he wanted to improve his political prospects.

It is difficult to imagine a more awful charge that could be leveled at a President—or one that is more foreign to every instinct and principle of the President I served.

No such operation was ever ordered by President Carter, "tentatively" or in any other way. The idea of launching a second rescue mission was never seriously considered or discussed. A contingency plan was, of course, developed. We had to have some plan of action in case the Iranians attempted something that gave us no choice: trying and executing the hostages, for example. But even those plans under development bore little resemblance to the invasion scenario described by Anderson. They were actually more akin to the surgical rescue operation that had failed in April.

Most importantly, conditions never arose that were even remotely consistent with the use of any military option and no order that was in any way similar to the one reported by Anderson was ever issued by the President or anyone else in the American government. The above statement is attested to by the President and Vice-President, the Secretary of Defense, the director of central intelligence, the Chairman of the Joint Chiefs of Staff, the director of the National Security Agency, and the President's adviser for national security affairs.

Anderson continues to insist that his columns were accurate, despite those denials from every senior official that would have been involved in such an operation.

It is significant that those denials came after the column was published. Anderson made no attempt to check with any of the above-mentioned officials before he wrote, a highly unusual, not to say unethical, action that can only be explained by the fear that such sweeping denials by the highest officials of the government would cause even the most complacent of editors around the country to question the veracity of his columns and perhaps reject them as preposterous.

At least one editor did just that. Struck by the fact that Anderson's initial column contained no reaction from either the White House or the Pentagon, Executive Editor Bradlee of the *Washington Post* called Anderson to find out why. Anderson's response, according to Ben Bradlee, was, "They would just lie."

Fortunately, that was not good enough for the *Post*. Bradlee tracked me down in New York at the convention. I told him I could issue a blanket denial immediately because I was being kept abreast of developments in the area. I also offered to back it up by putting him in touch with any other official he wanted to talk to from the President on down. He thanked me for the offer, but said he had asked Anderson for the documentation, which he claimed to have, that supported the astounding charges. He would wait to see what Anderson had to offer in the face of my denial before talking to other officials.

As it turned out, my supporting denials were not needed. As Bradlee and I were talking, *Post* Managing Editor Howard Simons and chief defense correspondent George Wilson were being denied access to any supporting documentation by Anderson. That was enough for Bradlee. The column did not run in the *Post*. Unfortunately for the President and for the credibility of journalism, it did run in hundreds of other newspapers around the country, as did the five columns on the same subject that followed.

Since the charges leveled by Anderson were false, there are two logical possibilities: Anderson was given forged documents to support what he wrote, or he has no documents to prove his allegations at all.

In a phone conversation with me during the preparation of this book, he said that he might have destroyed some of his supporting documents because recent court decisions making such material subject to subpoena in lawsuits "made it dangerous to keep that sort of thing lying around." He also said that in some cases he and his subordinates had only been "shown the documents" but had not gotten copies of them.

In an exchange of columns on this subject in July of 1983, prompted by information developed during the "Briefing-gate" scandal, I challenged Anderson to make what evidence he had or could come up with available to the National News Council, a group of distinguished journalists established in 1973 to review charges of inaccuracy against journalists. The council has both a commitment to and a flawless record of protecting sources. As this book went to press, that investigation was still under way.

One of the reporters involved in attempting to check out Anderson's charges would soon have direct personal experience with the disinformation campaign. In mid-August of 1980, George Wilson of the *Post* was contacted by a man who refused to give his name, but claimed to work for the CIA. For several weeks, this anonymous source tried to sell Wilson a variety of stories, all damaging to the Carter administration, and all supposedly based on classified information and documents. One described a CIA study, supposedly done as part of the planning for the April hostage rescue attempt.

According to Wilson's would-be tipster, this study predicted that one half of the hostages would be killed in the rescue attempt. Wilson was interested. The rumor that such a study existed had been floating around right-wing political circles for months. I remember hearing it repeated by an anonymous caller on a Washington talk-radio station in the first few weeks after the raid. Here was a chance for Wilson to find out once and for all. He told his caller that he would need something more substantial than just an anonymous voice over the telephone before he could write a story.

In mid-September he received through the mail the something more he had requested: a copy of what appeared to be a CIA study of the rescue operation, dated March 16, 1980, entitled "Oplan Eagle Claw Loss Estimate." The document predicted that 20 percent of the hostages would be killed or seriously wounded during the assault on the embassy compound, another 25 percent during the effort to locate and identify the hostages, and 15 percent more during their evacuation to the waiting helicopters.

Wilson's reaction was what Anderson's should have been. Wilson confronted the Pentagon with the information he had and demanded a response. It was not long in coming and it was unequivocal. Frank Carlucci, who was then deputy director of the CIA and later became Deputy Secretary of Defense in the Reagan administration, was the man who had supposedly ordered the study. He responded to Wilson in writing: "I have been unable to find anything in this alleged CIA document that is either accurate or which approximates any memorandum we prepared."

Wilson was convinced by Carlucci's denial and a CIA analysis of the forged document that listed a series of specific errors and inconsistencies, including the use of the wrong code word. No story about the bogus study ever appeared in the *Post*.

Shortly after the *Post*'s decision, Defense Department spokesman Tom Ross gave information on the disinformation attempt to CBS Pentagon correspondent Ike Pappas. Pappas thought it was a good story. He checked with Wilson and confirmed the specifics. But CBS was unable to find time for it on the evening news. Pappas was forced to do a piece for radio only.

But that was not quite the end of the matter. Two months later, Jack Anderson reported that he had learned of a secret CIA study that had predicted 50 percent casualties among the hostages from the April rescue attempt.

One of the most vicious ploys of the disinformation campaign was launched by members of the Madison Group in early September. Allegations were spread by Republican staffers on the Hill that David Aaron, deputy to National Security Adviser

Zbigniew Brzezinski, had been responsible for the arrest and execution of a valuable American spy in the Soviet Union.

The charges were false, and were eventually proven so, but not until after the election, and not before seriously disrupting the legitimate activities of one of the President's chief national security aides.

The ploy was successful in provoking a full-scale investigation by the Senate Intelligence Committee and in leaking word of the supposedly secret investigation to several news organizations, including the *New York Times*.

The initial reaction of the *Times* was questionable. Despite the lack of evidence to support the allegations, and the knowledge that a story on the investigation that mentioned Aaron's name could do great harm to his reputation and to the administration, a story identifying Aaron was published.

A few weeks later, on September 23, the *Times* became convinced that it had been used in a smear campaign and blew the whistle on those who were putting out the fabricated and terribly damaging information, naming names and describing their tactics. Those responsible for the Aaron smear were members of the Madison Group, and by that time their liaison with the Reagan campaign was in full operation.

One week later, Daniel Schorr, senior correspondent for Cable News Network, concluded an in-depth analysis of the affair in the *New Republic* by describing the attack on Aaron as "a classic piece of covert action [that] left the desired taint of suspicion."

Schorr was more correct than he knew. A few months later a book called *The Spike* was published. Written by Robert Moss and Arnaud de Borchgrave, two notorious right-wing publicists, it was an entertaining and thinly disguised polemic against center-left foreign and defense policies. Its thesis was that those involved in making and promoting such policies were not only wrongheaded and naïve, but probably Russian agents as well.

By way of illustration they described the "blowing" of an American agent in the Soviet Union by a high official in the Carter administration. The circumstances in their account were little changed from those contained in the false charges against Aaron. The character in their book was named Peter Cummings, and he was the deputy director of the National Security Council in the Carter (Connor in the book) administration.

* * *

A few weeks later, the Madison Group attempted to sell another fabricated story to Lesley Stahl, White House correspondent for CBS News. Lesley received a call from John Carbaugh, at the time on the staff of Senator Strom Thurmond of South Carolina. (He would later serve on the Reagan transition team for the Defense and State departments.) Carbaugh claimed to have information that demonstrated both the lack of will and the inconsistency of the Carter administration, and of the President in particular.

U.S. intelligence services, said Carbaugh, had compiled information that led us to believe that the Soviet Union was conducting nuclear weapons tests that were either right at or in excess of the limit established by the signed, but still unratified, test ban treaty. (Both sides had informally agreed to abide by the limits pending ratification, and the United States was honoring this commitment.) There had been considerable discussion, which reached the NSC, about how we should respond to this potential violation. One option was to conduct a test that was right at the limit ourselves to show that two could play at that game. The problem with such tests is that neither we nor the Soviets are able to monitor them precisely enough to know with certainty whether tests close to the limit are slightly over or slightly under.

Up to this point, Carbaugh's account was reasonably accurate. But then came the kicker. He told Stahl that the President had finally been persuaded to authorize an American test near the limit as a warning to the Russians. But he had given the go-ahead only with reluctance and after a great deal of pressure from the few "realists" in the administration. Preparations for the test had gone forward, the warhead had been set in place, and the actual countdown had begun.

Carbaugh even provided Stahl with the classified code name for the test and the technical name for the type of warhead that was to be tested.

Then, said Carbaugh, the President got cold feet. At the last minute he canceled the test, saying that upon reconsideration he was not prepared for a confrontation with the Soviet Union on this issue. The cancellation resulted in a rather significant waste of money, severe demoralization among those involved, and increased Soviet contempt for the resolve and constancy of the U.S. government.

It was a hell of a story, if true. Stahl filed a memo with her superiors at CBS. Word came back that if she could confirm what she had been told, it would lead the broadcast.

In contrast to the behavior of Anderson in similar circumstances, Stahl made an effort to do just that. She had by coincidence an interview with Zbigniew Brzezinski the next morning. When it was finished and the cameras were turned off, she asked Brzezinski about what she had been told. He apparently focused on the parts of the story dealing with possible Soviet violations and consideration of a possible American response, which were true. The situation was further complicated for both Stahl and Brzezinski because the subject was highly classified. Both were, as a result, talking around sensitive points rather than directly to them. In any case, Brzezinski's response seemed to Stahl, perhaps understandably, to be a confirmation of Carbaugh's entire account. She left the interview feeling that she had a blockbuster of a story, now confirmed at the highest levels within the White House.

Later that afternoon, after her story had been written and graphics prepared at CBS, Stahl called David Aaron, Brzezinski's deputy, with whom she had a longstanding professional relationship, and who was practically a neighbor in northwest Washington's Colonnade Apartments. The purpose of the call was primarily to check the technical terms used in her account. Stahl readily admits that she is no expert in nuclear weaponry, much less the jargon that is associated with this rather arcane field.

To her surprise and consternation, Aaron became extremely agitated, claiming that the story was wrong in every particular except for its claim that we were concerned about Soviet tests and were considering a response.

Stahl, in light of her conversation with Brzezinski, which Aaron did not know about, was also upset. She told Aaron that the story was going to lead the news that evening, and that she found his denial less than convincing. He invited her to come to his office immediately, and asked a National Security Council expert on such matters to join them.

After some discussion that appeared to be going nowhere, Aaron realized that he would have to take Stahl into his confidence to a greater extent than he would have liked to prevent the false and damaging information provided by Carbaugh from being transmitted to the millions of Americans who watch CBS News each evening.

Stahl reluctantly agreed to allow the conversation to go off the record, which meant that she could not report anything that she was told, but could use the information as a basis for making her own judgments about the situation.

Aaron then proceeded to explain that the President had never authorized a near-the-limits test, much less as a response to the Soviet provocation. There had, however, been a scheduled test, well within the limits, involving the type of warhead and with the code name given to Stahl by Carbaugh. That test had, in fact, been canceled late in the process—although not after the countdown had begun. The reasons for its cancellation were, and still are, classified. However, they were technical in nature and did not involve Soviet-American relations, the test ban treaty, or even the President. He had not even been involved in the decision to cancel because it was not a policy matter.

By this time, airtime for CBS was less than ninety minutes away. To her credit, Stahl informed the Washington bureau that her show-leading piece should be canceled. It was replaced by a report on Afghanistan. All she eventually got out of the exercise was a short story that ran on a hostage special late that evening, reporting that the United States was concerned about possible violations of the test ban treaty and was considering action to take in response.

This account is significant for two reasons:

First, and most obvious, it provides a striking contrast between the behavior of a legitimate news organization when presented with questionable information and the behavior of Jack Anderson in similar circumstances.

I often had my differences with CBS and with Ms. Stahl, as other sections of this book make clear. In this case, however, CBS and Ms. Stahl did their job well. They blocked an effort to gain partisan advantage through the use of the media to spread disinformation.

The second point relates to that disinformation campaign and specifically to this element of it. The story that was presented to Stahl was not in the category of amateurish rumor mongering. It was a sophisticated blending of fact and fiction, classified and unclassified information. It contained paraphrases of actual comments made by the President during National Security Council deliberations, taken out of context and applied to matters that were not even under discussion at the time.

To construct such a story required an intimate knowledge of tightly held information. Only someone who had attended that meeting, or who worked closely with someone who had been present, would have had access to the comments from the President. The other thing required was, in my opinion, even more important: a willingness to use the most sensitive national security information for partisan political purposes, to construct lies on that basis in an attempt to discredit the President and the government of this country.

THE HIGH COST
OF DECEIT_____

In addition to the moral repugnance of behavior like that of the sources for the nuclear test story, there are several practical considerations involved. Dealing with an incorrect story that involves classified information is one of the most difficult tasks in press relations, particularly when the false story has been constructed with an intent to deceive.

In almost every case, one is faced with a choice between telling a reporter more than he or she should know, or allowing a false and usually damaging story to run. Reporters, perhaps understandably, are no longer willing to accept a flat denial, without explanation, as sufficient reason to drop a sensational story. Part of that is due to the not very admirable reluctance of journalists to discard an exciting story, but an equally large portion of the blame has to be laid on government officials who use the "I can't tell you why it's wrong because that's classified" response to kill stories that are accurate. There are also officials who want to kill stories because they are politically embarrassing, not because they would damage national security.

That government practice is terribly destructive of the proper relationship between government and press. Worse, it erodes the willingness of journalists to protect legitimately classified information. The eventual consequence is that the public's confidence in government is eaten away.

At the risk of sounding self-righteous, I must say that using the "It's classified so you'll have to trust me" response to avoid political embarrassment was not among my sins. Nor, so far as I know, was it practiced elsewhere in the administration. Although I am sure that other officials were, on occasion, as sorely tempted as I.

Unfortunately, the present administration has not always been so resistant to temptation. It is ironic that those who speak most loudly about the need to protect state secrets, and make the most elaborate plans for doing so, seem to be the most willing to undermine that very system—not only by using sensitive information for partisan political purposes, but by using the trust-me response to protect the political interests of the administration rather than the security interests of the nation.

Such an incident took place while this book was being written. If reporters can be believed when they talk about their own feelings and attitudes, it resulted in an unhealthy climate of distrust between the National Security Council operation in the White House and the press.

The encounter occurred during the week of February 13, 1983, on a matter that was highly sensitive from a national security and a political perspective. What did and did not happen in the days that followed sheds light on an aspect of the press-government relationship that makes both sides uncomfortable, but neither can avoid.

The story involved the movement of AWACS (a highly effective command and control aircraft) to Egypt and the nuclear carrier *Nimitz* to the south-central Mediterranean. The sensitive aspect of the story, at least from a national security standpoint, was not the movement of ships and planes. The *Nimitz* had filed routine notices to airmen and mariners that described its general direction and destination. The AWACS with their distinctive radomes were clearly visible from public roadways near their Egyptian bases.

What administration officials wanted to keep secret was the reason for the deployments: they had learned of a planned coup against the government of Sudan that was to be supported by Libyan air and ground forces. In that context, those involved with the American operation had a number of legitimate national-security concerns.

Premature disclosure that the plot had been discovered might trigger the coup before the Sudanese were prepared to deal with it. Intelligence agents who had infiltrated the conspiracy might be endangered. If disclosure caused the coup to be aborted, key conspirators might flee before they could be rounded up.

On Tuesday, February 15, Pentagon officials learned that John McWethy, ABC's defense correspondent, was on to the military deployments and their connection to the Qaddafi-sponsored plot. McWethy was asked to hold the story for twenty-four hours and to soften some parts of it. He agreed.

The Pentagon notified the White House of the discussions with McWethy as a matter of course, and because President Reagan would need to be prepared to deal with the subject at his press conference on Wednesday night.

On Wednesday morning, officials at the White House decided to try to get the story delayed for another day. Apparently they wanted to make sure the President—who had not demonstrated great facility in handling complicated and sensitive matters at previous press conferences, and whose polls showed him to be vulnerable on the "trigger happy" issue—would not be faced with the subject at his press conference. (Since ABC had the story as an exclusive, they would certainly not blow their scoop by asking about it at a press conference televised by all three networks.)

Whatever their motives, the people in the White House, National Security Adviser William Clark and his deputy Robert McFarlane, failed in their efforts to kill or delay the story. ABC ran it on Wednesday's evening news.

In defense of the administration, it should be said that there is nothing inherently wrong with a request that a story be killed or delayed for national security consideration. It happens all the time. On two separate occasions during the hostage crisis, stories that would have endangered American lives were held in response to requests from the administration.

First Amendment absolutists sometimes argue that journalists have no responsibility for the consequences of their stories, that their only duty is to find the truth and publicize it. That sort of malarkey ignores the responsibility of journalists, as citizens, to help protect, or at least not to damage gratuitously, the system that allows them to exist. Perhaps more seriously, it also ignores the likelihood that the extensive privileges enjoyed by the press will not long survive if the public becomes convinced that those privileges do society more harm than good.

Contrary to reports at the time, the *Nimitz* story was not a plant designed to make the President look tough. In fact, the political concerns at the White House at the time were exactly the opposite. Their polls were showing that the President's greatest vulnerabilities were in appearing too warlike and too eager to use military force. In fact, the story was not even a leak, in the sense that that term is generally understood. McWethy had stumbled on the fact that there was a Libyan buildup of military forces on the Sudanese border while working on another story. He had learned of the AWACS deployment by chance, from an acquaintance who had a friend whose husband had been sent to Egypt with the planes.

Both Mr. Clark and Mr. McFarlane refused to discuss their actions on this matter, either on or off the record. However, the other evidence available suggests that what they did, or tried to do, was both improper and not very smart.

In the first place, they neglected to consult the White House Press Office, an error roughly equivalent to the press office's attempting to handle a coup in the Congo without checking with the NSC. As a result, their contacts with ABC were handled in a way that undermined their desired effect and promoted distrust and skepticism.

When the government asks a news organization to delay or kill a story, it must usually be willing to explain why. In this case, Clark and McFarlane refused to do so. They also refused to identify particular parts of the proposed story that were troublesome, choosing instead to claim that the entire report was wrong, which ABC knew to be false, because the story had been confirmed the day before at the Pentagon.

If specific reasons for the request cannot be given, the government has nothing to rely on but its credibility. This administration does not have an abundance of that commodity. Stories have been flatly denied that later turned out to be accurate. One such instance involving the role of American intelligence-gathering activities during the Falklands crisis caused a White House staffer to resign in protest. Mr. McFarlane exacerbated the problem by denying specific portions of McWethy's story that had previously been confirmed at the Pentagon.

McFarlane also violated another basic rule of such endeavors by telling ABC on Wednesday morning that no other news organization was working on the story. (It is standard procedure to warn a reporter whose cooperation is being sought if he is about to be scooped.) McWethy found out a few hours later that the *Wall Street Journal* was ready to go to press with the story and that the NSC knew it.

In the final irony, White House officials were apparently so preoccupied with killing the report that they failed to prepare the President. His response at the press conference was so fumbling and inaccurate that it gave even greater prominence to the story. One official involved in the process says that the President's answer was based on guidance prepared several days earlier to deflect routine questions about AWACS and *Nimitz* movements. Indeed, were it not for the rather astounding leeway the press allows this President on such matters—the excuse generally cited is that he is not intentionally lying, he just does not know—the patently false elements of the President's response might well have become a story in their own right.

The potential consequences of all this go beyond a generalized feeling of distrust between press and White House. It is possible, perhaps even likely, that ABC or one of the other networks will one day come to administration officials with a story that could do significant damage to national security if it runs as is. The officials may not be able to completely explain why the story should be killed or altered. If on that day ABC goes ahead and damage is done, whose fault will it be?

Certainly ABC will be at fault because they will have made a decision that turned out to be wrong, a mistake for which the country suffered. And it is vitally important that the news organizations be held responsible for the consequences of their mistakes, even in the presence of extenuating circumstances. That tendency of journalists to duck any and all responsibility for their errors just because someone else made mistakes too is one of the serious weaknesses of the profession.

But the administration will also bear a portion of the blame because they had, for purposes of political convenience, eroded that element of trust between reporter and government official which is the ultimate and most important protection against the disclosure of damaging national security information by the news media.

THE DEAL
THAT NEVER WAS_____

I n late October of 1980, the Reagan campaign's disinformation
effort struck again, and again with considerable success. An
"impeccable source" connected with the Reagan campaign
told Rowland Evans, of the famous—or notorious, depending on
one's point of view—team of Evans and Novak, a rather startling
tale. It would also have been big news, if it had been true.

According to this anonymous individual, President Carter's
legal counsel, Lloyd Cutler, had just returned from Geneva,
where he had met secretly with a high-level Iranian official. This
meeting was the culmination of weeks of secret diplomacy involving direct negotiations as well as intermediaries.

Cutler's trip, according to Evans's source, had resulted in a
"deal to exchange American hostages for military equipment vital
to the Iranian war effort against Iraq." The arrangement was "almost certain of fruition." It was timed to bring the hostages home
just prior to the November elections—an event that Carter was
"hopeful" would help him to win reelection. This infamous deal
had been "sealed with a handshake between Lloyd Cutler and the
Iranian emissary" at the Geneva meeting.

That October surprise the Republicans had been screaming
about on an hourly basis since the campaign had started was now
about to become a reality, and it was a tawdry sellout of the nation's interest and honor, as they had been warned it would be.
Evans and Novak were so excited by what their GOP source had
to say that they filed a "bonus" column (one in addition to their
regularly scheduled series) for release on October 31, four days
before Election Day.

In their column, they described in some detail the humiliating terms of the "deal." Those terms were *somewhat* similar to *some* of those eventually negotiated three months later in January of 1981. They also were related to *some* of the general categories that were indeed under discussion at the time. But what did not appear anywhere in the column were the elements of the final deal, or of the discussions taking place at the time, that were favorable to the United States.

Had the actual agreement been as described by Evans and Novak, it would have been seen, justifiably, as "rewarding terrorism" and paying "ransom," the very characterizations suggested by the column.

The truth was that Cutler had not been to Geneva since the spring, when he had gone over to discuss the Olympic boycott. He had never met with any Iranian officials. Nor was he playing a direct role in the hostage negotiations. Nor had he done so for months.

There were negotiations in progress at the time, but they were well short of success and were highly classified.

We could flatly deny the report, but we could not deal with specific areas, at least not on the record, without endangering the progress that was being made. Our predicament was almost certainly understood by the person who planted the story. There was no way, for example, for us to say, "Yes, we are willing to release the frozen Iranian assets as part of a final agreement, but only if there are also arrangements (as there were in the final agreement) to make sure that legitimate claims against the Iranian government are properly adjudicated and paid." To have done so would have moved the extremely sensitive and precarious discussions from the private to the public level, and almost certainly would have ensured their failure.

These discussions had actually begun on September 10, when an Iranian named Sadegh Tabatabai contacted us through West German Foreign Minister Hans-Dietrich Genscher. Tabatabai said he was authorized to work out the release of the hostages. Our sanctions—the blocking of trade, prohibition of financial transactions, freezing of assets, and the like—according to Tabatabai, had finally convinced even the clerical hardliners that the crisis would be ended.

The message relayed through Genscher also contained new

Iranian proposals that were significantly more reasonable than anything we had seen in the past, although they were still quite general and not acceptable to us. As proof of Tabatabai's bona fides, the message said that the Ayatollah Khomeini would shortly make a public statement confirming the terms set down in the secret proposal.

Two days later, the Ayatollah did exactly that.

Deputy Secretary of State Christopher was subsequently dispatched to Europe, ostensibly to consult with our allies on how we should respond to a Russian buildup on the Iranian border, which had in fact taken place, but also to meet secretly with Tabatabai in Bonn.

The meeting in Bonn was encouraging. Tabatabai stated that he would return to Tehran and make a favorable recommendation to his superiors on the Revolutionary Council and to Khomeini himself. Unfortunately, before he could get back Iraq invaded Iran, and the Iranian leadership turned its attention to the prosecution of that war, which was going very badly for them at the time.

We were determined to pursue the promising initiative, but our initial guarded optimism had now largely vanished. The discussions were not revived for more than three weeks. In mid-October, Christopher was again sent to Bonn to meet with Tabatabai. Again the results were encouraging, but we also learned that the matter would have to be resolved by the Majlis, the Iranian parliament or what passes for one. We had seen possible agreements come apart over that issue before, and we were not particularly optimistic that this crowd was capable of doing anything constructive.

Although we certainly wanted the hostages home as soon as possible, we had all but given up on the idea that it could be accomplished before the elections. Not only that, we were going out of our way with the Iranians to downplay the idea that this was a crucial date for us, figuring that such an assumption on their part would only make them more unreasonable.

If the release of the hostages was to take place at all, the momentum for it would have to come from the Iranians. It was essential that they accept this fact and act in accordance with it.

In that sense, the Evans and Novak column was not only

wrong, it was potentially damaging to the very tentative negotiations under way. It was also damaging because Genscher was extremely sensitive about keeping the discussions secret for fear that the role of the West German government would become known. The Germans' concern was understandable since they still had diplomats and other nationals in Iran. They feared, and rightly so, that militants who did not want to see the hostages released might take revenge on the nearest available German. The Germans also had reason to be worried, although this was a lesser factor, about the violently radical groups of every conceivable political persuasion in their own country.

To make matters worse, neither we nor the Germans were at all certain that the Iranian initiative was backed by, or even known to, all factions in the government. (Nothing else that had taken place on this matter had failed, sooner or later, to become a bone of contention in the domestic struggle for power in that chaotic and benighted country.)

The fact that the initiative had come from individuals associated with the clerical faction and had apparently been legitimized by Khomeini's speech gave us some hope for its eventual success. However, Tabatabai and the other Iranian officials involved had made it clear from the outset that their lives would be in danger if knowledge of their role became public prematurely, leading us to the conclusion that there were still powerful factions in Iran that were interested in seeing the crisis prolonged. Our conclusion was confirmed when the Majlis debate on the new Iranian proposals began and a large number of its members boycotted the session in an attempt to keep any favorable action from being taken.

It was obvious too that the Soviets had a vested interest in preventing a settlement. We were at great pains to keep them from knowing that discussions were under way. Given their excellent intelligence operations and that of their allies in Iran, they would soon find out which Iranians were involved and who the leaders were. The Soviets had shown in the past a willingness to take extraordinary measures, including assassination, to promote their interests, even when they were bound to be the prime suspects. In this case, the death by gun, bomb, or knife of a few more Iranian officials could have been easily arranged with no likelihood that anyone except us would have suspected that the

KGB was involved. And even we would have been in no position to prove it.

Thus it was that a column that was politically damaging—the thrust of the Evans and Novak report was that the Carter administration once again was subordinating diplomacy and our national honor to political considerations—was also potentially dangerous to the national interest.

In my mind the offense was compounded by the fact that the story had come from an individual connected to the Reagan campaign who clearly had an ax to grind. Not only did Evans and Novak fail to warn their readers that their source was potentially tainted, they also failed to make any effort to check with the Carter administration officials who were supposedly key players in the events.

My relations with the two columnists had never been good and were in an abysmal state by this point in the administration. (That I allowed this to happen was, despite the provocation, one of my more damaging mistakes—but more about that in the concluding chapter.) Under the circumstances, it is perhaps understandable that neither Evans nor Novak called me to check out the report.

However, Rowland Evans and Lloyd Cutler, the purported central figure in the story, had been friends for years. They had in fact seen each other socially on at least one occasion while the column was being written. But Evans never asked Cutler one word about the column. Nor did he even check on whether Cutler had been to Geneva or out of the country during the past several weeks. (Cutler had not, of course, and certainly would have said as much if asked, thus providing a strong warning that there was something wrong with the story. Had Evans been willing to be precise about the basis of the column, he would also have been told that there was virtually no chance on earth that any agreement could be reached, much less the hostages released, before Election Day.)

Evans would later say that he had said nothing to Cutler because he did not like to ask questions of government officials that he knew would force them to lie. He also stressed that the individual who had given him the tip was in a position to know what he was talking about. Evans may have been sincere in his reasoning, but in this case (as he candidly admits) he made a terrible mistake, resulting in the publication of a story that was totally false.

There was heavy irony in all of this, which may well be obvious to the reader by now. However, out of an abundance of caution, let me make it explicit.

The publication of this dangerous and inaccurate story involved two columnists who had been charging for months that the President was using the hostage crisis for political purposes, and that he was sacrificing our national interests out of a desire to win reelection.

The source of the column was someone closely connected with the Reagan campaign, an organization that had been trumpeting the same allegations to anyone who would listen. Their message to journalists and to the public was "Watch out, Carter is going to do anything it takes to get those hostages back before Election Day, and he is just the sort of scoundrel who wouldn't think twice about selling the country down the river if that was what it took."

Yet it was the Reagan partisan who used the hostage crisis for political ends. It was his planting of a false story to help his candidate in the elections that endangered the national interest. And it was Evans and Novak who failed to check the story adequately— whatever their reasons—and thus allowed themselves to be used in a way that was both political in its motivations and potentially damaging to the nation's welfare in its effect.

(It should be noted here that Evans believes to this day that his source did not intentionally mislead him. If Evans is right, that simply means that his source was himself misled. It only pushes back the question of who did the fabricating at least one step. It defies all logic and experience to believe that a story this detailed and complicated was the result of an honest mistake or misunderstanding.)

Nor is that all. There are more serious implications to this episode, particularly in light of the other disinformation efforts by the Reagan campaign and evidence that campaign officials were obtaining and using highly classified material in this political effort.

Evans's confidence in his GOP source is significant. Although I am not a great fan of the Evans and Novak column—we commonly referred to it in the White House as "Errors and No Facts"—I am inclined to believe him when he says that he considered that source to be "impeccable." Although they are not above the use of innuendo and insinuation to make a point that is less than well documented, they are not in the habit of stating flatly that such and such a major event will take place unless they are reasonably confident that they will not be embarrassed by subsequent events.

As I told the President at the time, "They aren't sweethearts, but they ain't stupid.'

Had they simply wished to damage the President and cast a shadow over a hostage agreement that *might* take place prior to the election, they could easily have done so without going so far out on a limb.

Since Reagan campaign officials had no legitimate access to the highly sensitive information about the Tabatabai discussions, they must have been able to convince Evans and Novak that they were well plugged in through sympathizers inside the government.

Given the revelations almost three years later that the Reagan campaign was indeed running an intelligence operation involving several former CIA and FBI employees, the purpose of which was to spy on the American government, it is not surprising that Evans and Novak could be convinced that the story they were handed was accurate.

The implication here is clear. Once again, the Reagan campaign was involved in attempts to breach the security system of their own government—a security system that they profess to hold in the highest regard now that they are in office. Once again, sensitive intelligence data that in the wrong hands could have damaged American interests and even endangered lives were being passed through nonsecure channels, bandied about a campaign headquarters, and even handed out to journalists. And once again, the motive for this irresponsible, if not illegal, behavior was a consuming desire to win an election.

ON THE TRAIL
OF THE MOLE_____

Y ou'd think people would learn, but all the historical evidence is to the contrary. In the early summer of 1983,
when the advance copies of *Gambling with History*, a book
by *Time* magazine's White House correspondent, Laurence Barrett, began to arrive in selected Washington homes and offices, not
everyone dropped everything they were doing to read through it.

One who did was *New York Times* White House correspondent Steve Weisman. He found that the book, though far from
unfriendly to the Reagan administration, contained a rather startling revelation: the Reagan campaign had had "a mole in the Carter camp," who stole a copy of President Carter's briefing
notebook for the 1980 presidential campaign debates.

The book also revealed that some of the highest officials in
the Reagan administration had been involved in, or at least knew
about, the theft: Jim Baker, now White House chief of staff, who
presented the material to David Stockman, now budget director.

Stockman, who was involved in his own campaign for reelection to his House seat, had been called in at the last minute to
play the role of Carter in Reagan's debate rehearsals. (Stockman
had apparently been a showstopper as John Anderson, his former
employer, in earlier debate rehearsals.)

Stockman, who knew the notebook was stolen property, was
delighted and found it to be a great help in preparing for his performance.

When the debate was over, again according to Barrett, the
Reaganauts were pleased to note that the notebook "had included

every important item Carter had used on the air except one: his reference to his daughter Amy, in connection with nuclear arms control." (An awkward aside that hardly required a response. Only in retrospect have the public and the press come to realize that Amy's concern about Ronald Reagan and nuclear weapons was altogether justified.)

Finished reading, Weisman began calling around to former Carter officials in an attempt to check the story further. When he called me on Monday, June 6, 1983, I could hardly believe my ears, being among those who had not yet delved into Barrett's tome.

I told him what I remembered about the briefing book and the preparation process and suggested that he call Pat Caddell and Stuart Eizenstat, who had been more directly involved in the preparation of the debate briefing book than I had.

Later that afternon, I called ABC's White House correspondent, Sam Donaldson, to let him know that I thought there was an interesting story in the works. (I was and still am an employee of ABC News, although not as a reporter, and try to pass along tips on stories whenever I run across them.) Donaldson's reaction, which was decidedly unenthusiastic, should have tipped me off to the way the world of White House coverage had changed in two years.

I should not have been surprised when no story appeared in the *Times* the next day, or the next. I was. When Weisman called again on Wednesday morning, I was more than a little curious about what he would have to say. What he said, rather sheepishly and with evident embarrassment, was that the *Times* had "decided there's no story in it."

Surely he was kidding. What really had happened was that the *Times* had assigned an investigative team to make sure their first story was a good one. Weisman was just trying to get a rise out of his old sparring partner. Right?

Dead wrong. America's newspaper of record, the organ that had put a highly dubious accusation by two indicted felons against Hamilton Jordan on the front page, did not think the fact that two of the most powerful figures in the government had admitted receiving and using stolen campaign materials was newsworthy.

I expressed my feelings on the lack of news judgment at the

Times—including the unnecessarily provocative observation that it was now easy to understand why they got their socks beaten off on Watergate—and asked whether he minded if I did something on the story in my Sunday column, given the extraordinary expression of indifference at his paper. He said he had no objections and hoped someone would pursue the matter.

It was amazing that the Reagan people would engage in such skulduggery in the aftermath of Watergate, which some of them had observed at close hand. But the initial reaction of major news organizations was even more mind boggling: a collective shrug and yawn.

Barrett had filed his "dirty trick" story with *Time* in February of 1981, but it was "crowded out by other news." (*Time*'s pages were presumably filled with more important items for the next 108 weeks.)

Time's Washington bureau chief, Bob Ajemian, suggested that Barrett's original story may not have been written "with enough conviction," but had no explanation for the lack of follow-up. Indeed, Ajemian said he actually could not remember ever seeing the item, and did not think it important enough to go back and check on what had been filed or what had happened to it.

The *New York Times*, which had spent two days fiddling with the story and then discovered there was no news in it, decided that some sort of story had to be run after Weisman told his bosses that I intended to pursue the matter. So they settled on burying the story instead of killing it. The day after my second chat with Weisman, the *Times* managed to squeeze in four paragraphs on page B-10.

As it turned out, there was no need for the Timesmen to worry. The *Washington Post*—prompted by my call to one of their White House correspondents who was well connected with the Reaganauts to check on what he knew of the story—gave it six paragraphs on page 16, reflecting little effort and less interest.

I could not help but think about what would have happened under similar circumstances in days gone by. Suppose Hamilton Jordan and Bert Lance had been accused of using material stolen from the Ford White House to prepare Jimmy Carter for the 1976 debates—not admitted, mind you, which was what had happened here, but just been accused. It would have been Katie, bar the door. The whole smelly mess would have been on page 1 from day one. Investigative teams would have been assigned to ask pointed, unpleasant questions. Answers that smelled of evasion or inconsistency would have been treated with derision and contempt. Editorial demands for the White House to make a clean breast of it and jettison the sleazy Georgians, who were undoubtedly responsible for this outrage, would have run throughout the land. I would have been able to talk about little else at the daily briefings, barring war in Europe or a *Hustler* interview with Billy, until the truth had been dug out.

But the press seemed to have forgotten how that process worked. In just twenty-nine short months the fourth estate had reached that blessed realm where lions become lambs, typewriters are beaten into plowshares, and rear ends in the White House become objects for kissing rather than kicking.

One of my political friends offered, merely as a topic for speculation, the question of how the press would have reacted to a revelation that Carter's campaign, or Reagan's for that matter, had been stealing and using private documents from the files of a newspaper or network.

After calling Baker, Stockman, and Communications Director David Gergen—at Baker's suggestion—and becoming more convinced than ever that they were hiding something, I wrote a column setting out the facts as I knew them and raising questions that seemed to need an answer:

What other dirty tricks had the Reagan campaign perpetrated?

The fact that the notebook had been stolen not from the campaign headquarters but from the White House, and that less than a dozen people were ever authorized to see it, strongly suggested that the person who took it had access to other information, even more valuable to the Reagan campaign. Was it logical that he (she?) would risk copying and sneaking out a three-inch-thick notebook but ignore more important information that could be passed over the telephone?

Who else in the Reagan campaign was involved? Was the mole paid in cash? With a job? A pat on the head?

I had learned of Gergen's involvement from Baker, but Baker failed to mention CIA Director William Casey, whose name would surface in a few days. Both Baker and Gergen claimed to have only the vaguest recollection of the whole incident; both said they could not even recall who had handed them the notebook. I was presumably expected to believe that it had been left under someone's pillow by the tooth fairy.

In his book, Barrett described how Baker agonized over the "ethical dilemma" presented by the stolen notebook. But when I talked to him, he said he had not even tried to find out who was responsible so he could make sure it did not happen again.

Then there was the question of whether candidate Reagan knew he was using stolen material.

Baker, Stockman, and Gergen swore they never told their boss anything. That was frankly hard for me to believe. It still is.

In October of 1980, both camps viewed the debate as the most crucial event of the campaign. At that point, pollsters for both sides saw the race as a dead heat. It defies all reason and logic that Mr. Reagan would never be told that what he was hearing from Stockman in the rehearsal was the genuine stuff, not just someone's best guess of what Carter might say.

Finally, there was the legal question of whether the Ethics in Government Act required an FBI investigation of the theft and use of this material.

I asked Zoe Baird, a lawyer who had served as associate counsel to the President during the Carter administration and who had been involved in the drafting of both the original legislation and the amendments that were passed in 1982. Her answer was "Yes!" (The attitude of the Reagan Justice Department, which may be the most politicized since enforcement of the nation's laws was in the capable hands of John Mitchell, would, not surprisingly, turn out to be a rather contorted "We don't think so.")

That question bears directly on whether it will ever be possible to learn what actually happened. An administration that is willing to lie, to baldly claim not to remember even when the lack of recall defies belief, can make it almost impossible for the press, by itself, to dig out the facts. A legal investigation, however, puts greater pressure on those involved. If they can be shown to have lied, they face possible legal action and an almost certain setback in their career path.

The *Post* ran my column on Sunday, June 12, even though it

took a swipe at the paper's news judgment. To say that the earth failed to move would be an understatement. The press continued to exhibit the same studied indifference, except for Steve Goldberg, a young reporter from the Richmond papers who decided to pursue the matter on his own time, despite the active opposition of his superiors.

The only other significant response was a call from *Time* bureau chief Ajemian to accuse me of trying to cause trouble between him and Barrett. I assured him that was not my intent, expressed regret if that had been the effect, and asked if he had found the time to go back and look up the original *Time* story (the one that had been crowded out by other news for better than two years). He had not.

The entire matter would have died right there, without any doubt, except for a couple of young staffers on Congressman Donald Albosta's Subcommittee on Human Resources of the Committee on the Post Office and Civil Service. They decided the committee had jurisdiction, since government employees were almost certainly involved, and determined to do what they could to get to the bottom of it.

Their opening move was simple, straightforward, and brilliant. Albosta sent polite, nonaccusatory letters to Gergen, Baker, Stockman, and Casey, asking them to tell what they knew about the business. (Casey was included because he had been Reagan's campaign manager and also because, as one staffer put it, "If there was anything sleazy going on, you had to figure William Casey was right in the middle of it.")

The sending of the letters received routine and distinctly uninspired coverage. But when the answers came out, twelve days later, the worm turned.

The written responses from Baker, Casey, Stockman, and Gergen were notable for their studied ambiguity and inconsistency. They were the first hard evidence of a frightening amnesia epidemic that was sweeping through the ranks of senior administration officials. In short, the responses raised far more questions than they answered.

Chief of Staff James Baker said he had received "a large, looseleaf, bound book that was thought to have been given to the Reagan camp by someone with the Carter campaign" from William Casey.

CIA Director Casey said he had "no recollection" of ever seeing or hearing of any such thing.

Baker said he had passed the notebook to the "Debate Briefing Team" headed by David Gergen, now White House director of communications. Mr. Gergen said he did not recall ever seeing or receiving it or anything else that might have come from the Carter campaign. (A statement he shortly retracted with profuse apologies when "hundreds of pages of Carter documents" were discovered in his files. They had, he said, been misfiled under "Afghanistan.")

Stockman, who admitted to being the last person to have the briefing material in his possession, said he could not find one page of it now. He guessed that his staff had thrown it all away, along with all the rest of his debate preparation papers, when he moved to the transition office—a surprising and unfortunate, or fortunate, loss to history, depending on one's point of view.

Here was another claim that was hard to swallow. In 1980, David Stockman was a bright young congressman with ambition, but uncertain prospects. Because of his past association with John Anderson, he got a chance to impress the GOP nominee at the first debate rehearsals. His boffo performance there earned him a call-back when the Carter-Reagan debates were finally scheduled.

Thanks in part to his efforts, Reagan won the debate and the election. From little-known congressman to president-maker in less than sixty days, and Stockman throws away every scrap of paper, every note and memo associated with his meteoric rise to national prominence. Buy that one on faith, and I'd like to talk to you about some aluminum siding.

The other point that Mr. Stockman was careful to include in his letter to Albosta was a statement joining all his colleagues in attempting to downplay the importance of the material he had used. (Even officials who could remember almost nothing else, and who were not even sure they had ever seen any documents, were by this point quite positive in their public statements that whatever was there was of no significance.) Indeed, the dismissal of the purloined material as "not important," "inconsequential," and dealing only with "matters of public record" had clearly become the administration's principal line of defense.

It was based on the hope that the press could be convinced that there was nothing there worth wasting any time on, a not unreasonable strategy at the time, given the indifference with which reporters had greeted the first disclosures. (When I spoke to Gergen, Baker, and Stockman three days after the *New York Times* began working on the story, and the day after the *Post* published its brush-off article, they said it was the first call they had taken from a journalist on the matter.)

Realistic though the strategy may have seemed, it was decidedly peculiar from an ethical standpoint. It is not generally considered much of a defense for one charged with stealing a horse to claim that the critter turned up lame and never was much use to anybody.

In addition to the contradictions and improbabilities contained in the letters themselves, there were also conflicts between descriptions of the material in earlier comments, made before the controversy began to heat up, and those contained in the letters.

The latest characterizations were clearly designed to promote the idea that this was some sort of general collection of Carter administration accomplishments or past statements by the President. However, Mr. Stockman and Frank Hodsoll, the second-in-command of the Gergen debate team, had stated earlier that the documents were in "question and answer" format—a significant distinction since the Carter debate book had been placed in that format only in the final stages of its preparation.

Stockman had also said earlier that the Carter material was the only thing he used to prepare himself for his role in prepping Mr. Reagan for the debates, a statement that appeared to be in conflict with his later attempts to claim that none of it was of much use.

The total lapse of memory extended, of course, to how the material got to the Reagan campaign in the first place. None of the big four had any idea. But their subordinates had not been so circumspect. Miles Martel, a consultant called in for the debate, was told by Hodsoll that the Reagan campaign got the material "from someone inside the Carter campaign," and Martel says "the word 'mole' might have been used."

The release of the letters put on the record an official admission that briefing material taken from the Carter White House had been used by senior officials in the Reagan campaign—that and a tangled web of inconsistencies and obfuscations.

That was a problem for those who were interested in getting at the truth. But it was also the beginning of a problem for the White House. The letters from Albosta had given Casey, Baker, et al., a chance to provide a reasonable and convincing explanation of what happened. Instead of laying the matter to rest, their cagily worded responses and selective recall actually quickened interest and heightened suspicion.

As a result, the Justice Department, which had been dismissing the matter as simply a case of "political disloyalty," had to change its tune. It was changed as little as the political appointees in the department felt they could get away with, but it changed. An investigation was even begun.

In an effort to keep the thing from getting out of hand, however, the investigation was not classified as one under the Ethics in Government Act, thus avoiding the question of a special prosecutor.

However, if the investigation, which is still under way as this is being written, is aggressively pursued, administration and former campaign officials will face specific and detailed questions about what they did and what they know, backed up by legal penalties if they fail to tell the truth.

Mr. Reagan, who dodged questions for a week and then contradicted himself and his aides, will be asked precisely what he knew and when.

Professional and personal relationships between Reagan campaign officials and White House employees that raise the possibility of a pattern of political espionage will need to be explored.

How vigorous the investigation would in fact be now moved close to the top of the list of questions on the Briefing-gate list. Fortunately, since the Reagan Justice Department is not known for vigor in its examination of senior officials, congressional investigators from Albosta's committee began asking the same intriguing questions.

The most visible response to the release of the letters, however, was a complete change in attitude on the part of the press. Reporters all over town began scrambling to catch up with a story that had been lying under their noses for two weeks. The few journalists who knew a little about what was going on were deluged with calls from anxious journalists wanting to be "brought up to speed on this briefing-book business." Young Mr. Goldberg's work, which had been virtually ignored by his own paper, became the basis for lead stories in major newspapers and on the networks.

All of this put me in an even more awkward position than I had been from the start. As a clearly interested party, I was hardly the best, or most credible, person to be writing about the matter. I had overcome those concerns at the outset with the rationalization that, awkward position or not, no one else was going to raise the questions that needed to be answered.

Once I had written, however, it did not seem appropriate for me to become engaged in flacking the story all over town to other journalists. Although this is not an unheard-of practice among columnists, I had considered it to be questionable at best when I was in the White House, and I was hesitant to engage in it now.

After discussing my dilemma, which also included a request from the committee to talk with them informally, with several experienced journalists whose reputations for integrity are unquestioned, I decided that I should respond to questions if asked by either journalists or congressional investigators, but should not initiate such conversations myself.

It seemed a reasonable and defensible posture, but I was prepared to take some heat, particularly from the administration and from the commentators who automatically sprang to its defense. As it turned out, I got a great deal less than I expected, primarily because the ethical dilemma question became focused on another, much more experienced and widely read columnist.

George Will had long been a Reagan booster. It was even known that he had been present during some portion of candidate Reagan's preparations for the debate with President Carter. What was not known until the week of June 26 was that he had participated in the preparations for the debate and that he had known Stockman was using material taken from the White House.

Newsweek magazine had asked Will what he knew on June 10. He did not get back to them until almost a week later. That is perhaps understandable, since he knew his response was bound to cause him problems and no doubt hoped, as did his friends in the White House, that the whole thing would blow over.

What is not understandable is how *Newsweek* then behaved.

No politician would have been allowed to duck such an interesting question for a week unless he left the country.

Even worse, once the magazine had the answer, they still wrote nothing on it. Only after Will revealed his participation on network television did they decide to give it a few cautiously written paragraphs.

Not surprisingly the reaction among journalists was intense. The world of Washington journalism divided into supporters and defenders of George Will. It was a wonderful sight to behold: the fourth estate, for one of the few times in its history, was being forced to examine its less than pristine ethical petticoats in full view of the rest of society.

It would have been more of a pleasure for me, of course, had I not been involved in an awkward conflict myself. In recognition of my own delicate position, I stayed out of the debate.

However, since this book is about the press, and one of its themes is the reluctance of journalists to subject their colleagues to the same scrutiny that they apply to the rest of society—and since I am now in the commentating and columnizing business myself—here it is.

I cannot on general principles defend the idea of a columnist actually participating in the campaign of a candidate he is writing about, even though he deals in opinion and his preferences among candidates are well known.

The difficulty comes in the potential conflict of interest between the responsibilities of any journalist, even a columnist, to his readers, and to the requirement of confidentiality when stepping into the midst of someone's campaign. And it was precisely such a conflict that faced George Will the moment he saw the Carter briefing books lying on David Stockman's kitchen table.

What he saw was a big story. No matter what he thought of the ethics of the matter, there was absolutely no doubt that this was news. Had it become public in the final ten days of the campaign just prior to the debate, the press coverage would have been substantial—to say the least.

I have no doubt that if George Will, or any other journalist, had discovered that the Carter campaign was involved in such shenanigans, he would have written about it without delay. I also have enough faith in Will's integrity, despite the criticism expressed here, to believe that he would not have ignored behavior in the Reagan campaign that he would have condemned in another.

The difficulty was that he did not "discover" the information. It was handed to him by campaign officials who clearly saw him not as a journalist but as a partisan. To have ratted on them then would have been a terribly low blow.

Indeed, I must say that under those circumstances I would not have written about the stolen briefing books either. It may not be proper for a journalist to assume the role of campaign adviser, and I definitely believe it is not. But if you assume that role, you must play by its rules. To fail to do so would only compound bad judgment with treachery.

While the commentators in the press were debating the proper relationship between pundits and pols, the reporters were beginning to uncover some rather interesting information. The most startling part of which, to me at least, was that the Reagan campaign had set up a network of former and active military officers, intelligence agents, and FBI agents to spy on the American government—to gather up classified information for use in a political campaign.

A former admiral, David Garrick, revealed to the *Washington Post* that he had personally supervised an operation in which retired and *active duty* military officers reported to the Reagan campaign on the movement of American ships, troops, and aircraft. The purpose was to obtain forewarning of any sudden break in the Iran crisis, but the effect could have been calamitous.

Suppose there had been the need to mount another rescue attempt. Say we had gotten word that the hostages' lives were in imminent danger, for example. As we sought desperately to get our forces secretly in position for such an attempt, reports on our movements, from American military officers no less, would have been flowing into the Reagan headquarters in Alexandria, Virginia, over open and nonsecure phone lines.

Anyone familiar with the level of sophistication and the sheer amount of electronic eavesdropping in Washington will tell you that these reports might just as well have been phoned directly to the senior KGB operative at the Soviet embassy.

Had we been forced to make such a move, the chances are

great that the Reagan campaign's political espionage operation would have unwittingly tipped off the Russians, plus several other not always friendly nations with high-quality intelligence services. The Russians then would have only needed to pass the word to the Ayatollah's thugs, and the American rescue team would have been ambushed and either slaughtered or captured.

The other interesting angle to surface was the Kennedy connection. On July 3, CIA Director Casey made public the name of one Paul Corbin, as a person who had supplied him with some material, although not the Carter briefing books. Casey's revelation was prompted by Corbin's boasting to an associate that he had given documents from the Carter administration to Casey. The associate had passed the information on to Jim Baker, who was in the midst of a conflict with Casey over their contradictory responses to the subcommittee—Baker saying that he had gotten the material from Casey, and Casey saying that he had not.

Casey apparently chose to make Corbin's name public before Baker or one of his allies did so. Casey also took the opportunity to say that he had checked with Corbin, who had stated that all he ever gave Casey were some speech suggestions for Reagan from former Robert Kennedy aide Adam Walinsky.

Corbin is interesting because he is and has been for years a faithful political retainer of the Kennedy family, first doing what one former co-worker described as "Chuck Colson" work for Robert Kennedy, then working for Teddy. He worked in the 1980 Kennedy campaign against Carter and then almost immediately went to work for Reagan. Both he and the Reagan people have been rather vague on exactly what sort of work he did.

What makes Corbin even more interesting is his relationship with Steve Smith, Kennedy's brother-in-law and chairman of Senator Kennedy's 1980 campaign. Corbin, according to one who has worked with both, "is a wholly owned subsidiary of Steve Smith. He would never make a political move without Smith's permission."

That raises the question of whether the Kennedy family encouraged their people to work for Reagan and whether they knew what sort of work they were doing. It also raises the possibility that the warning from Republicans in the Congress that a thorough investigation of political espionage in 1980 would embarrass some prominent Democrats, including the senior senator from Massachusetts, may not be a red herring.

At this writing, the investigations by the FBI and the Justice Department are still in progress, and what they will ultimately turn up is largely a matter of speculation. However, it is possible to make a couple of educated guesses.

The focus of both inquiries has shifted from the original interest in briefing books containing material on domestic policy matters to concern about the penetration of the national security area, and to the role of present and former national security and intelligence officials.

Former Reagan National Security Adviser Richard Allen has revealed that he received information from Zbigniew Brzezinski's morning reports to the President, which contained extremely sensitive material. (Allen says what he got was "innocuous," but that makes no more sense than the early, and since disproven, claims that the briefing book material was merely a list of administration accomplishments. Why would someone with access to these reports and bent on helping the Reagan campaign win the election pass on only useless portions?)

Robert Gambino, former chief of security for the CIA; Stef Halper, son-in-law of former CIA Deputy Director Ray Cline; Cline himself; Max Hugel, whom William Casey tried to install as head of covert operations at the agency; and a good handful of former CIA and FBI employees have all been linked with the Reagan campaign's intelligence-gathering operation.

Evidence is reportedly in the hands of both the committee and the Justice Department that ties both Casey and James Baker more closely to documents stolen from the Carter operation than either has been willing to admit publicly.

If there is a smoking gun, or more likely a large, smelly dead cat, to be found, it will almost certainly be in the national-security intelligence-community area.

That is in many ways regrettable. Any such revelations will inevitably be used by both political extremes to support their pet theories. On the right there will be charges that the press and the Congress are just out to beat up on the CIA and the Pentagon again. On the left some will use the information to do just that. And without doubt the public images of both institutions, which have just recovered from the damage caused by the revelations of the mid-seventies, will be hurt.

Should that unfortunate circumstance come to pass, however, it will be important to remember that behind it all were individuals who served in the military and the intelligence agencies, putting partisan politics ahead of the oath they swore when they took those jobs.

It will also be worth remembering how close we came to never knowing at all that anything might be amiss. The press, which has proven many times over its ability to turn a molehill into a mountain, this time nearly succeeded in doing just the opposite.

The most dangerous bias in the press, as I said earlier in this book, is not political but economic—news judgment based on what is interesting and salable. In this case, most of the powers that be decided initially that stories about dirty tricks against the Carter administration had no market two years later. That judgment may have been influenced by the generally negative attitude toward Carter that still exists among Washington journalists.

Whatever the reasons, the press yawned when it should have gasped. And the public almost missed the opportunity to learn of activities that may bear directly on the ethics of senior officials and the security of classified documents.

A
RECOMMENDATION_____

About two years ago, after a decade as a government spokesman and campaign press secretary, I accepted offers from the *Dallas Times Herald*, the *Los Angeles Times* Syndicate, and ABC News to try the columnizing and commentating business. It was a surprising decision to many who knew me well. During my years in politics I had often spoken even more unkindly than in the preceding pages of journalists in general and commentators in particular.

One friend and former colleague from those years said it was as though someone who had been a doctor for most of his adult life had suddenly decided to become a disease.

Another colleague and former friend was unkind enough to recall that I had often described columnists as the kind of people who view the bloody conflict from afar and then—when the fighting is done and the warriors have departed—come down from the hills to shoot the wounded.

But for me the temptation was too great to resist. I had never in ten years been able to get a columnist to write what I wanted the way I wanted it. Having failed to beat 'em, I figured joining 'em was a reasonable alternative.

Mostly though, I could not resist the opportunity to view this system of representative government and the grand game of politics from a more detached and perhaps more objective perspective. And it seemed only fitting that I try walking a mile in the shoes of those I had so often berated in the past. I was also well into the process of writing this book, or what eventually became this book, and it seemed that some practical experience on the other side of the fence would inevitably give me a better feel for the subject I was trying to address.

Some twenty months later, I am impressed, most of all, as I indicated at the beginning of this book, by the similarity between the problems that beset those in politics and those in journalism:

• Neither institution is held in particularly high regard by the American people.

• Both are always having to make decisions based on information that is woefully inadequate, which may account for some of the lack of public confidence.

• But the most striking and dangerous similarity is oversensitivity to criticism—that circle-the-wagons, us-against-them, everyone's-out-to-get-us reaction that sets in when the crap hits the fan.

I saw it, participated in it, and sometimes led it when I worked in the White House. There were occasions when it was justified—in Washington being paranoid does not necessarily mean you are crazy—but seldom did that excessively defensive reaction fail to do more harm than good.

I must say, however, that the inability to handle criticism is worse in the press than it is in government. It is not because of the quality of the personnel, since there appear to be an equal number of rascals and rounders in both institutions. It is because there is no established mechanism for rooting out and exposing ne'er-do-wells in the fourth estate.

In politics the opposing party, disenchanted factions within your own party, and most importantly the press are constantly looking for a chance to point a finger at error and incompetence. No remotely similar process operates to check and restrain journalists.

There is, to be sure, the occasional ombudsman. And there are publications, such as the *Columbia Journalism Review* and the *Washington Journalism Review*, that undertake serious analysis and criticism of journalistic issues and behavior. The problem is that organs of press criticism do not have the resources to undertake the sort of in-depth investigation that is commonly focused on wrongdoing in other institutions.

There is a vast difference between being criticized by *CJR* or by your local ombudsman and being pilloried in the lead story of a network news program. The censure of peers is not without some effect, but it can hardly be compared with being held up to disdain and ridicule before a good portion of the entire nation.

The fourth estate's hostile reaction to criticism, of virtually any sort from almost any quarter—and the corresponding lack of such criticism—is the most dangerous shortcoming because it, more than any other single factor, inhibits attempts to correct or at least alleviate all the other problems.

Or, to put it more positively, if we can deal with the lack of hard-hitting analysis and criticism in journalism, we will have taken a long step toward dealing with most of the difficulties caused by deadline pressures, inadequate information, greed, laziness, bias, and the like.

As I have traveled about the country over the past three years, I have had the opportunity to participate in more than my share of seminars and symposia on journalism, which I suppose tends to cut against my contention that journalists never listen to criticism. Certainly they never heard many kind words from me at such appearances, although there may be some question as to how well they listened.

In any case, I noticed that one of the most frequent topics at those gatherings was whether or not the press can be both competitive and responsible. I happen to believe that it can.

That belief does not place me in the same category as one of my Southern Baptist brethren who, when he wās asked if he believed in infant baptism, replied, "Believe in it, hell, I've seen it done!"

I have never seen what I am about to propose done, but I believe in it nevertheless.

Putting government in charge of establishing standards of accuracy and accountability for journalism is not the answer—except for some tightening of the libel laws, which is a subject for another day. But there is no good reason why the press should not shoulder the responsibility for cleaning up its own mess.

It seems to me that what journalism needs more than anything else is real competition—not just two strong, independent newspapers in every town, but no-holds-barred, take-off-the-gloves competition similar to what exists in politics.

If your competitor is a liar, or lazy, or cavalier with the truth, say so.

If the opponent makes a serious mistake, pounce on it, tell the world about it.

If you think your opponent may have made a mistake, find out. Don't just sit around waiting for an admission of guilt and an apology. Dig up the evidence and force the admission and apology if an adequate defense or explanation is not forthcoming.

If the *New York Times* accuses someone of wrongdoing based on flimsy evidence, why shouldn't the *Washington Post* or the *Wall Street Journal* or the *Los Angeles Times* feel an obligation to check into the matter and, if need be, set the record straight?

If ABC blows its coverage of a major story, thereby misinforming tens of millions of people, why shouldn't CBS and NBC and CNN accept the responsibility for answering the public's legitimate questions about what happened and why, and what is being done to keep it from happening again?

If it is news that a member of Congress is sleeping with his or her secretary, or snorting coke, maybe it ought to be news if a nationally known journalist is doing the same thing.

And wouldn't it be great if the same people who write those magazine pieces about "The Ten Dumbest Congressmen in Washington" would turn one out on "The Ten Dumbest Columnists in Washington"? Now that would be a horse race. It would take a photo finish to separate the top five.

More seriously, if the public has a right to know, and they certainly do, when an official who helps make energy policy owns oil company stock, isn't there a similar right, even need, to know if a journalist who is reporting or commenting on that policy— and is thus in a position to influence its ultimate content—has a similar conflict of interest?

Are there powerful media figures who do report and comment on matters in which they have a direct financial interest? The answer is that for the most part no one knows—not even the people who run the newspapers and networks and newsmagazines.

Members of Congress and senior executive officials are required to disclose the amount and sources of outside income, but most journalists are not, not even to the news organizations for which they work.

An informal survey of the three networks and four of the nation's largest newspapers determined that not one has any serious procedure for checking on the financial entanglements of their editorial staff. Their reporters could be on the payroll of an oil company, a labor union, the KGB, and the Moral Majority for all they know.

It is common knowledge that the better-known reporters, editors, network anchors, and columnists make large sums of money from the lecture circuit, commanding fees much larger than the average senator or congressman could hope to draw. Are these journalists speaking to groups who stand to profit from what is written or said through the public media by their honored and honoraria-ed guest speaker? The answer again is that no one knows. But someone should. In fact, we all should.

I see no reason why, as a matter of policy, news organizations ought not to require those who cover the Congress or the White House or an executive branch department to make the same type of financial disclosures as the people whose shoulders they are looking over.

The journalists could even use the same forms as the public officials, thus sparing their hard-pressed companies any undue financial burden. The completed forms could be turned in to the same office that receives them from the government officials— which office I feel sure would make public the reporters' financial statements at the same time that they released those of the government employees.

If there is something questionable in one of those reports, let the press be responsible for finding out the facts of the matter and letting the public know.

Why, in short, shouldn't journalists apply some of the same standards of ethics and competence to their colleagues as they do to powerful figures in the rest of our society? Then that old saw about the public having the right to turn the dial, or buy another paper, if they do not find what they are getting acceptable, would mean something.

Politicians sometimes argue that respect for government is eroded when journalists treat those public servants who behave decently as badly as those who do not—thus reducing substantially the incentive to be decent. And there is some truth to the allegation. In journalism, the problem is the reverse: those who behave and perform badly are as immune to censure as those who do not. The result is the same.

Most of us learned at some point in our youth that the best way to get people, including ourselves, to do right is to introduce into their minds and hearts a healthy fear of what will happen to them if they do wrong. That fear of retribution is what is lacking in the fourth estate.

As a consequence, journalism suffers by protecting rascals who ought to be ridden out of town on a rail. And society suffers as journalism squanders the credibility it must have to lay the wood to knaves and fools in other walks of life.

Our democratic political system cannot survive without a strong, aggressive, and responsible fourth estate. If that is lost, sooner or later everything else we treasure in the way of civic values will also be gone.

I do not believe that the free press in this nation is an embattled institution. Nor do I believe that the First Amendment is in danger of imminent repeal or evisceration. Indeed, I suspect that some of the talk about such catastrophes is designed precisely to discourage serious journalists from taking a discriminating look at the behavior of some of their so-called colleagues.

While I was writing this book, I attended a round-table discussion on press coverage of the Iran hostage crisis, involving former government officials and several of the more thoughtful and responsible representatives of national news organizations.

After those of us from government had spent several hours denouncing one inaccurate and irresponsible story after another, indictments that were often undisputed by the journalists, I asked in frustration why, if they agreed that these stories had been inexcusable and that some of the people responsible for them consistently failed to meet even minimal journalistic standards, why did they not rise up in indignation and warn the people of the country that they were being fed claptrap by charlatans?

One of the most decent and thoughtful of all the national journalists I know replied, with evident sincerity, that he had long ago concluded that he had to "protect the Jack Andersons of this world" to make sure that good journalists were also allowed to do their jobs.

I believed then, as I do now, that the truth is exactly the opposite. If I turn out to be wrong in my belief that a free press is relatively secure in this country, it will not be because of constructive or even destructive criticism from some former press spokesman such as myself. It will be because the fourth estate has contracted that disease which is most certain to be fatal to any major institution in our society, a massive and continuing loss of public confidence.

That cannot, must not, be allowed to happen. And it is the responsibility of everyone who understands the importance of a free press as well as its shortcomings to do what they can to see that it does not.

WHITE HOUSE FLACKERY _____

I t may well seem presumptuous to some for a press secretary who managed to take his boss from almost 80 percent in the polls to a landslide loss in four short years to be passing out advice on the White House press secretary's job. It may well even *be* presumptuous.

On the other hand, it is the fighter who has taken the most punches who knows most about how to roll with them. And it well may be that the press secretary who has stepped in it the most has learned something about how to spot it before you put your foot down.

In any case, I could not close this book without delivering myself of some observations about the job I held and, despite it all, enjoyed for four years. Those observations have been seasoned by the three years that have passed since I left the job. But to be honest, they have not changed a great deal.

The press secretary's job remains in my mind, as it was the day I walked into the West Wing, the pick of all the staff positions in the executive branch. Nowhere else does a person have the chance, indeed the necessity, of being involved in so much so fast. Cruise missiles, breeder reactors, snail darters, well-head prices, and undocumented workers: they all come across your desk sooner or later. Usually two or three at a time. And often when you least expect it.

Furthermore, the daily briefings and constant contact with the press provide an outlet for pent-up energy and aggression. Other White House operations seldom have a chance to confront directly their client-adversary group. But the press office is toe to toe with the source of at least a major portion of a President's difficulties each and every day.

People in other offices may be frustrated by their inability to confront directly teenage unemployment, or Soviet adventurism, or wasteful energy practices, but in the press office, the problem is right there where you can get your hands on it, at least figuratively.

That incessant sparring, arguing, and cajoling, and the constant review of the stories that result, give the feeling, perhaps illusory, that you are actually doing something that has an impact.

A good portion of the pleasure and stimulation that comes with the job is derived from the tremendous amount of talent and experience that you can call upon. Pick up the phone and you have within seconds someone who knows about as much as any human being alive on almost any subject you can name—particularly if the federal government has some stake in it, and there is not much that does not fall into that category.

One principal frustration of the job is the lack of time to take advantage of all those bright people in the government, who are just waiting for someone to ask their advice on some subject to which they have devoted a lifetime.

Besides the lack of time, sometimes it is just not knowing who and where they are. On more than one occasion, I spent more time trying to find the right people to talk to than it took them to tell me all I needed to know.

The other great pleasure is dealing with the press. Despite all I have said in the preceding pages, and I take back not a word of it, reporters are as interesting a crowd as will ever darken the gates of hell. For all their shortcomings, and despite their tendency to run in packs and fly like blackbirds in the same direction at the first loud noise, they are a great breed of individuals.

Getting to know the reporters who are covering the White House, plus some of the more important ones on major beats such as Defense, State, Justice, and the like, is high on the list of a press secretary's responsibilities. Having to talk to a reporter whom you really do not know about an even moderately serious matter is an unnerving experience, and rightly so.

I had long finished my first lengthy conversation with Walter

Pincus of the *Washington Post* on the enhanced-radiation warhead, or neutron bomb as it came to be popularly and inaccurately known, before I found out that as a congressional staffer he had been deeply involved in and generally hostile to such projects. Had I known all that when I picked up the phone to return his call, I might not have been able to do much to head off the frenzy that his paper subsequently went into over the weapon, but I certainly would have been in a better position to try.

On more than one occasion I got myself into trouble sitting around chatting with local reporters I had never seen before during presidential trips. I was interested in getting to know them, instilling a little goodwill, and relaxing. They, as I kept reminding myself to no avail, were interested in getting a story out of the President's visit that went beyond the usual speech handout and schedule routine. Failing all else, a semi-outrageous comment from the White House press secretary would do just fine.

Indeed one of the frustrations of the White House press job, as opposed to the same position in a governor's office, is that there are so many reporters and so little time that it is difficult to get to know as many individually as one would like.

However, a word of caution is in order on the "getting to know" point. In the main, it is probably not a good idea to develop close friendships with reporters who are covering the White House. Rarely will anything good come of it. Sooner or later, if both are doing their jobs, one will be required to do something that makes the other's life exceedingly unpleasant, if not downright painful.

That creates a certain amount of tension under any circumstances. But if you find yourself saying not just "How could that SOB do such a thing?" but "How could that SOB, who I thought was my friend, who sat in my house, bounced my children on his knee, and drank my good whiskey, do such a thing?"—the trauma is much worse.

One of the perversities of the job is that it requires spending a great amount of time with people who are impressed by the amount of time you spend with them, and keeping a certain distance from those who are going to do their jobs without consideration for social amenities. I suspected at the time, and have confirmed since, that it is the latter that you will prize as friends over the long haul.

Beyond that, there are some general rules of procedure, which are worth about as much in specific situations as general rules usually are, but probably merit setting down as points of departure, if nothing else.

Number one on the list has to do with bad news, which is to say most news. As the old saying goes, "When in doubt, get it out." No matter how smelly it seems to be at first, it always gets worse as it ages.

It goes against human nature to stand up of your own free will and volunteer information that is bound to cause nothing but trouble. More than that, it can be a delicate bit of business to try to convince others that you should go out and reveal something that is bound to be extremely painful for them.

Still, in nine cases out of ten, it is the only smart move. "Life," as several Presidents have said at one time or another, "is unfair." There is neither the time nor the resources in any administration to fight every fight, answer every challenge, and take every issue to the bitter end. When it is clear that the matter is either a loser or at best an unacceptably expensive close call, the smart thing to do is cut your losses. And the best way to do that is to lay the painful part out yourself, rather than wait for it to be dragged out.

The second most important rule, which has been alluded to earlier, is "Read the cables." Make sure you know what you are talking about before you go out and do verbal battle with the fourth estate. They can ask a dozen stupid questions and write an equal number of ill-informed stories and get away with it. One dumb answer that has to be corrected and explained later will cripple a spokesman for days.

It may appear that these first two rules are in direct conflict. That is because they are. In fact, the tension between being timely and being accurate is the principal cause of mental instability among press secretaries and what keeps the job interesting.

One factor that adds to the difficulties of being accurate is the extent to which any spokesman must depend upon others for information. The deputies and assistants in the press office spend much of their time collecting information for the press secretary to use in briefing the press. And they in turn must depend upon dozens of other people scattered about the White House and Cabinet departments for what they feed to the press secretary.

There is sometimes a tendency among political and policy people to tell a press secretary not what actually happened but what that particular person thinks ought to be said about what happened. It is deadly. By the time the gleanings of several deputies and assistants in the press office are put together and the press secretary has injected his own bit of information and right reason, the resulting presentation to the press can be badly off the mark—unless it is based on nothing less than the cold, hard, usually unpleasant facts.

Usually that inclination to tell you *what to say has happened* rather than *what actually has happened* is motivated by nothing more sinister than a desire to be helpful. Everyone wants to be a press secretary, figuring he can do the job at least as well as whoever happens to hold the position at the time—often with some justification.

However, it is occasionally the case that bad information is delivered to the press secretary, not out of an innocent desire to be helpful, but because the person being questioned is trying to cover his rear end. Such situations, although I found them to be extremely rare, lead to another general principle for press secretaries.

It is most helpful for the press secretary to have, or to be thought to have, a reasonable amount of clout within the administration. This means, in the final analysis, clout with the President. The purpose is much like that of the Strategic Air Command. You do not really want to use it, but you want to have the right people worried that you might. In short, it can be helpful at times for others to be more worried about what will happen to them if they lie to you than if they tell the truth.

While we are on the subject of clout, another word of warning is in order. It is a mistake, I think, for the press secretary to invest any major portion of whatever influence he has in the interminable squabbles over policy and programs.

In the first place it is a squandering of resources. The press secretary's job is the press. Dealing with that crowd will more than consume whatever resources of influence and persuasion the press secretary can command.

The other reason for staying clear of the policy fights is that they can be enormously destructive of the sort of internal relationships that a press secretary needs to do his job. The extent to which he must depend on accurate information from others has already been mentioned. Getting that information can be more difficult than it is ordinarily if the press secretary and the person he is calling for help have just been on opposite sides of the bloody fight involving the matter under discussion, especially if the press secretary's side has won. The policy person at the other end of the line may be tempted to say, "Well, you seemed to know so much about it when you were arguing against my recommendation—why don't you figure it out yourself."

On the occasions when the press secretary's views have not prevailed on an important and controversial matter, he still has the duty to explain and defend the President's decision to the best of his ability. If he is known to have lobbied vigorously against the option chosen, there will inevitably be some who wonder deep inside whether or not his heart is really in what he is being paid to do. Occasionally that might even include the President.

The most important reason for ducking the policy conflicts has to do with an answer I sometimes give, only partially in jest, when asked about the qualifications for the press secretary's job: "The ideal person would be a confirmed dilettante with a touch of ham."

Dilettantes with a flair for performing in public are not necessarily the best policy advisers. The principal characteristic of press operations in the White House, on both sides of the podium, is superficiality. The name of the game is skimming off the cream, seizing on the most interesting, controversial, and unusual aspects of an issue. Some understanding of and feel for the nuances is required, but it is usually just enough to get by.

Policymaking by the press secretary is roughly equivalent to a government run by a directorate of newspaper editors—or Mr. Reagan.

There is another side to keeping clear of policy battles, because the press secretary needs to have an understanding of what they are about. Those private conflicts may end up in the press the next day. Even if they do not, they provide a preview of the questions and arguments that you will face once the decision is made and the policy is announced. You often need to be at the meeting, but not as a full-fledged participant.

Furthermore, press secretaries, as I sometimes argued to little effect, are human beings, too. Your judgments may be superficial, but they are there nevertheless. On occasion, they may be every bit as good as those of the experts, who sometimes miss large issues in their fascination with nuances. There are times when a sense of right and wrong and propriety demand that you not remain silent.

In such cases, general rules and standard operating procedures have to be set aside. Even so, it is still wise to weigh in very early, when there is a chance to head off a bad idea before it attracts widespread support, or very late, when the number involved in the discussion has been narrowed and you can make your argument directly to the President.

I must confess that I violated the rule against getting into policy fights more often than I should have. However, I did so less frequently than was generally thought on the outside. (Fortunately for the President and the Republic, it is clear in retrospect that my advice was almost always wise, compassionate, and sound.)

So far, I have been speaking of the press secretary's job as though there were general agreement on what it is. That is not the case. The scope of its responsibilities and where it stands in the White House pecking order have varied greatly from one administration to another, and even within the same administration. What is clear from the experience of the past thirty years or so is that there are a number of organizational arrangements that can be made to work, and none that can be guaranteed to work.

About the only function that is always identified with the press secretary is the daily briefing, which is unfortunate. That responsibility, important as it may be, is too time-consuming for the senior person in charge of press relations to discharge.

I make that statement as one who insisted on doing the briefings almost every day. It was a mistake that limited my effectiveness and, I think, hurt the President.

The problem was that I spent so much time on the day-today problems, reacting to crises, stomping out brush fires, and the like, that I sadly neglected the long-range aspects of the job: the planning and overseeing of a communications strategy for the President and his programs.

Although there is some tendency to devote an excessive amount of time to immediate problems (when you are due at the podium in thirty minutes, it is difficult to think strategically), that is not the crux of the difficulty. The fact is that handling the daily briefings is a full-time job. Though I am sure some would do better at finding time for the longer-term responsibilities than I did, I do not think it is likely that any single human would be able to do both adequately. That view, I might say, is generally supported by those who have gone before me, as well as those who have come after.

The answer is most assuredly not to try to split the briefing duties. Briefing is a seamless cloak, particularly when the going gets tough. How you handle a matter or a question or a reporter may depend a great deal on how you dealt with it yesterday or the day before. Reading a transcript will not suffice. Preparing for a briefing, if you have not briefed for a day or two, takes an inordinate amount of time. And when you stand up in front of the reporters you are still left with the feeling that you are not quite ready, a feeling that is usually accurate.

When there are two regular briefers, it is also inevitable that one will be considered the second-stringer. The determination of which one is so regarded may or may not have anything to do with the skill or the amount of accurate information that is transmitted. It may be personality, or titles, or age, or who is perceived to be closer to the President. Whatever the basis, the distinction will always be made, and it will usually be grossly unfair to the person dubbed number two. More important, it will inevitably limit his or her effectiveness, particularly in a ticklish situation.

Both the Carter and the Reagan administrations tried the alternating-briefers approach, and both wisely abandoned it.

The ideal solution, closer to what the Reagan administration has ended up with than to the one I devised, is a full-time briefer who occupies the press secretary's office reporting to a director of communications who has more general responsibilities.

I say "reporting to" for want of a better term, but the relationship would have to have a great deal of flexibility to actually work. The press secretary would still need direct access to the President, for appearance sake if nothing else. And he or she should also have a great deal of autonomy in deciding how a matter will be handled in the briefings once the basic policy line is set.

The director of communications, on the other hand, should take over the responsibility for one of the people who are often neglected in the rush and pressure of daily briefings—the President. The press office should play a much greater role in decisions relating to the President's activities than it does in most administrations. As I found to my dismay, there is simply not enough time for a person who is briefing every day to play that role adequately, even when others in the White House are quite willing to listen.

Speech preparation, scheduling, advance work, anytime the President is to appear in public or is deciding whether or not to appear in public: all these need a strong influence from the press office. But they do not always get it. The President is, after all, the focus of interest on the part of the journalists. It is ridiculous, but not uncommon, for a press secretary to neglect decisions affecting the President's personal actions because he has to get ready to explain why the Cabinet Secretary responsible for overseeing aid to the poor and downtrodden put a personal chef on the federal payroll, at a time when the President was talking about austerity and balanced budgets.

One part of the President's activities in which the press office has always played a major role deserves mention here: press conferences. Our commitment to hold two a month was foolish. A President simply has more important things to do with his time than prepare for two full-blown press conferences each month.

On an average, one every four to six weeks ought to suffice. As transmitters of information, they are vastly overrated. I often felt that the nation would have been better informed about what President Carter was up to had his town hall meetings been televised instead of his press conferences. Not because the citizenry asks more intelligent questions than the press, but because they ask questions about the things they want to know about.

However, there is danger in a President's waiting too long

between sessions with the press. He tends to lose his feel for the medium. His sense of an issue, which makes the difference between an adequate response and a good one, fades quickly.

Worse still, it is much more difficult for the President to prepare himself factually. There is no way for any human to keep at his fingertips all the information that might be needed in a thirty-minute press conference. Briefing materials are essential. But even the best briefing book cannot possibly remind or inform a President of everything of importance that has happened during a two- or three-month period. The danger here is that an adequate answer turns into a terrible one. This danger is particularly acute if the President tends to be, shall we say, detached.

There is also a public policy argument for presidential news conferences on a reasonably regular basis. The American people have a right to see how their Chief Executive and Commander in Chief handles himself under tough cross-examination, without benefit of a text that has been carefully polished and endlessly rehearsed. The ability to perform adequately in such situations is not the most important qualification a President should have, but it is well up on the list.

A President who is not quick enough to handle the unexpected question, or not sufficiently in command of the facts to construct an effective counterargument off the top of his head, will be at a serious disadvantage in dealing privately with foreign leaders and diplomats, not to mention the contending policy proposals of his own advisers.

Since Presidents, like all mortals, occasionally make mistakes, one especially ticklish part of the press secretary's job is deciding if and how to set the record straight. On the whole, I would suggest caution.

I probably tended to do too much fine tuning on matters that were of not very great importance in the great scheme of things. It usually boils down to a question of whether the mistake will receive greater attention if you correct it or if you leave it alone. And in most cases the answer is to leave it alone.

Even when the press does get excited about a presidential misstep, it usually does more harm than good for the press secretary to become excited, too. Most Americans are quite aware that our leaders are not infallible. They are inclined, I suspect, to be reasonably tolerant of honest errors—even to react in a way that is sympathetic to the President when the press gets too carried away on subjects that just do not seem that important.

When the press secretary comes out to correct the record, however, it sends something of a signal to the public that this must have been something serious after all. Otherwise why all the effort to straighten it out?

Nor is the press above attempting to goad a spokesman into correcting a statement by his boss for want of a better story, or just for the pure hell of it. Sam Donaldson of ABC was, and by all accounts still is, a master provocateur. On more occasions than I like to remember, he ended up with a story that was one part what the President said and five parts what I had offered later by way of explication. A wise press secretary is well advised to shrug off such attempts and tell Sam and his cohorts to do their damnedest with what they have.

Part of the problem here results from the image that some in the fourth estate have of themselves as guardians of the truth and protectors of the public against half-truths and weasel words from shyster politicians.

A portion of that job description is indeed a legitimate function of a free press. If a President makes a statement that is flatly wrong, particularly if it is self-serving, the press has an obligation to call that to the attention of the public.

But the press is not the other political party. The job of reporters is not to argue over which of several reasonable interpretations is the absolute and only one that should be considered as acceptable.

Oil deregulation, a cap on hospital costs, and the B-1 bomber may or may not be good ideas, but they are all reasonable options. The job of the press, it seems to me, is to accurately report the arguments on both sides and to try to keep them reasonably honest. It is most decidedly not the job of reporters to make the arguments for either side.

When journalists become confused about their proper role in life, it is generally best to ignore them and hope they will soon settle down. The last thing a press secretary is obligated to do is help them make their case against whatever it is that his boss has just said. If they want to play leader of the opposition, they should be forced to rely upon their own wit and ingenuity.

While we are on the subject of misbehavior by journalists, a word about dealing with the real brats in the group. Unfortunately for press secretaries, and I suspect for the nation, many of the brats also tend to be influential.

Power and prestige seem to have roughly the same effect on journalists as on South American colonels. They immediately begin casting about for someone's fingernails to pull out. Then they expect to be treated as gentlemen and accepted in polite company as soon as they have cleaned the bloodstains out of their dinner jackets.

Nevertheless, as I learned to my dismay, it is seldom productive to write off an important reporter or commentator just because he or she is a retarded adolescent. The price of not doing so can be extremely high in frustration and psychological trauma, but the cost of doing it can be even higher to the President.

With sufficient effort and a willingness to grovel before one's inferiors, it is usually possible to remain on civil terms with even the most obnoxious of the breed. (For one thing, the worst of the lot are usually columnists or commentators, which means that you do not have to deal with them every day.) You may not get but one decent column out of twenty in return, but that is one more than you would have gotten if you had dismissed them as entirely hopeless.

One way to lighten this particular burden is to make use of all those other White House staffers and government officials who want to play press secretary. Ask one of them to give you a hand with old so-and-so. With a little luck the two will develop a close relationship. In that event, if you have selected your intermediary carefully, you can also take satisfaction from the thought that the two probably deserve one another.

Despite all that, it may be permissible in a few, very special cases to tell one of these pompous pundits exactly what you think of him, his wife, his dog (when you can tell which is which), and what his mother did during the war. So you lose that one column out of twenty; sanity and self-respect have got to be worth something.

There is another group of journalists who are often considered, incorrectly, to be a great burden to the press secretary. Here I speak of the real, genuine crazies. (By "genuine" crazies I mean those whose mental disabilities go beyond megalomania.) These people represent a wide variety of fringe political views, factions, and circles. The males can usually be identified by their penchant for wearing leg warmers over their trousers. The females make a habit of biting their nails in place of cleaning them with a brush. Individuals of both sexes may appear at first glance to have only one eyebrow.

Contrary to popular opinion, these creatures were actually placed on earth by a compassionate Providence to assist press secretaries in time of trouble.

When you are nose deep in the mire of some difficult and potentially embarrassing affair of state, there is great comfort in knowing that just by pointing to the right person you can get such questions as:

"Why is the FBI harassing the Socialist Workers Party and trying to poison Lyndon Larouche's rat?"

"How many senior administration officials are former tri-lateralists and Bildebergers?"

"Why has the President stuck his finger in the eye of Israel?"

"Would the First Lady disown her daughter if she did/didn't have an abortion?"

With a little creativity, by the time you have finished dealing with an issue like one of these, the rest of the pack may have totally forgotten the line of questioning they were pursuing on Iran, inflation, or drug use among White House aides.

Nothing clears the mind and calms the soul quite like devoting a portion of the daily briefing to heaping abuse and ridicule on one of the bona fide berserkers in the press room—then coming back to your office, closing the door, and speculating over a cup of coffee on the proposition that life is not always unfair.

All of which leads naturally to the role of temper in the relationship between White House and press. There is indeed a place for it, although it is usually not the place where its exhibition would be the most satisfying.

When a reporter is wrong, and you both know that he is wrong, there are two basic approaches. The first is to appeal to a sense of responsibility and fair play. Unfortunately, evolution over the centuries has resulted in the atrophy of those character traits among reporters, in much the same manner as the legs on a snake have shrunk into two small internal bonelets entirely invisible to the casual observer. That leaves an impressive display of righteous indignation as the only, albeit forlorn, alternative.

The key is to create the impression that you are so angry that you just might do something extraordinary. It is important not to indicate exactly what you will do, since your options are severely limited. Some reporters are more easily intimidated than others. They will respond to the implied threat that no one in the White House will ever talk to them again and that their names will be stricken from the press Christmas party invitation list. The more seasoned veteran may actually suspect that you will send an anonymous letter to his wife about the stewardess in Denver, or to her boss about the administrative assistant on the Hill.

Whatever the reason, such outbursts occasionally work. In one instance during the debates over the Panama Canal treaties, two reporters from one of the wire services had compiled a story based entirely on lies from Hill staffers who were attempting to defeat the treaties. Their masterpiece contained allegations, all false, that officials from State, Justice, and the White House were involved in a conspiracy to hide and perhaps destroy intelligence material that had been subpoenaed by the Congress.

The story had moved on the wire, which is how we found out about it, since the reporters had made no attempt to check their "facts" with any of the administration officials whose reputations they were about to destroy. Fortunately, however, it was embargoed for the next day, and that gave us a chance to get it changed before it ran in thousands of newspapers around the country.

I called the officials involved to my office and got a quick briefing on their side of the story. In the meantime, the two reporters and their boss were on the way over. Once they arrived, I allowed the accused officials to lay out the facts without interruption from me. When they had finished and the reporters began to niggle over details without any attempt to defend the damning thesis of their story, I pitched a fit.

I will not bore the reader with a recitation of all the histrionics involved. Suffice it to say that they ranged from a vivid characterization of the kind of news organization that would move such a story without even listening to the other side, to suggestions on which libel lawyer my colleagues should retain the moment this meeting was finished, to a declaration that I would personally write and lobby for the inclusion of two paragraphs on this incident in the President's upcoming speech to the nation on the Canal treaties. My briefing on that speech would most assuredly include what I knew (which was nothing) about the personal relationships between the reporters and their sources that might have prompted them to file such a story without checking it.

For whatever reason, it worked. The offensive story was withdrawn and a largely innocuous one in the same general area, which few papers used, was filed in its place.

It may have been my performance that did the trick. The female member of the reporting team was later quoted as saying that I had stormed out of the office and slammed the door (true), and that I was so enraged that she feared I would do her physical harm (visions of the strangulation scene from *The Godfather* did cross my mind). It is equally probable, perhaps more so, that the story was withdrawn because the bureau chief, despite his lack of sympathy with the administration politically, was convinced that the story was indefensible and acted as bureau chiefs are supposed to act in such situations, but too seldom do.

Before leaving the subject of temper, two final points should be made. First, I must confess that my advice on this subject, as on much of what has preceded it, is largely a case of "Do as I say, not as I did." On the whole, I tended to get mad and showed it in situations where no good could come of it, and considerable harm was a serious possibility.

In a few cases, I exploded without checking the facts thoroughly myself and unfairly accused some journalist of being a liar, scoundrel, and mortal threat to the nation. On other occasions I said things that, while arguably accurate, could have gotten me in serious trouble had they ever appeared in print. That they did not is evidence that some snakes do have usable legs after all. In general, the positive effect of temper is enhanced if it is used sparingly. Just because it makes you feel better, or because the story in question is an offense against humanity and common decency, is no excuse for getting mad.

Finally, there is no more appropriate way to end a discussion of temper than with a word or two on humor. For that matter, what better ending could there be for a book about the press and the White House?

For someone such as I, given to unpredictable and sometimes irrational outbursts, humor was the balm that usually kept the wounds from festering. It prevented small problems and transgressions from becoming major incidents and bitter feuds on more occasions than I care to recall. Humor made it possible, on most occasions, for me and the reporters I worked with to let the shouting matches and harsh words be bygones and start fresh on the next morning or the next story.

For all of us, on both sides of the podium, it was often the last refuge and only sure defense—the ultimate recourse that enabled us to live with ourselves and, after a fashion, with each other.

Far from being out of place when there are portentous matters afoot, as some stuffed shirts would have us believe, humor is most desperately needed in precisely such circumstances.

How else can one shrink the swelling head, whether it sits on the shoulders of a press secretary, pundit, or President, without inflicting painful wounds and permanent scars?

How else can one keep the issues of ultimate import to a size that is manageable by the human mind and approachable for the human psyche?

What better way to end a confrontation when the stakes are large, both sides are adamant, and neither side is in a position to win?

A soft answer may indeed turn away wrath, but a humorous one can turn it upside down and inside out. Few of us can maintain a posture of belligerence or self-righteous indignation or offended innocence if we are laughing.

There are books filled with examples of political humor: the favorite anecdotes and stories that public figures recite on the stump or in after-dinner speeches. That has its place, but it is not exactly what I am talking about now. The humor that is most valuable in public life is that which is private or semiprivate: the exchange of quips from the Oval Office to the situation room to the press room that takes some of the charge out of the air and loosens the muscles in the back of the neck.

Those exchanges are essentially private, even when made in the briefing room, because they depend so much upon the mood and atmosphere of the moment for their meaning. They are almost impossible to translate for someone who was not there. Even for those of us who were, most of them are funny now only in memory.

Looking back over the transcripts of briefings and notes of meetings, I come across moments from reporters and officials followed by the notation "(laughter)" or "(prolonged laughter)." Not always, but in many cases, it takes a moment or two before it becomes clear what we were laughing about. One has to go back mentally and emotionally to what the moment was like, to the feel and smell of it all.

That is also true for much else that appears in those notes and transcripts. Most of it has meaning primarily in the context of a particular time and place. And not surprisingly, when I am trying to recreate that context, it is the points of humor that offer the quickest bridge back.

Looking back now, I regret, as much as anything else, that all of us did not laugh more at ourselves and the world around us. If there is one thing that Washington needs, it is the ability to see the amusing, even silly, side of much that is taken so seriously—primarily by people who want so desperately to be taken seriously themselves. The reason that happens so seldom, I suspect, is that deep inside the most pompous and self-important know very well how ridiculous they are. Their greatest fear is that the rest of the country will someday figure it out.

From my earliest days in the governor's office in Atlanta, I have been threatening to write a book about my experiences with the fourth estate. The theme, I always vowed, would be taken from one of those stories (probably apocryphal) that all state legislatures produce in great abundance.

For many years, one of the most bruising legislative battles had been over funding of the fire ant eradication program.

On the one side were arrayed the farmers and other agricultural interests for whom fire ants were no laughing matter. On the other, environmentalists and the like who did not have to deal personally with the ants, but saw nothing very amusing about Mirex, the chemical used to get rid of them.

The debate usually boiled down to an irreconcilable argument over whether the insects or the poison did more damage, and to whom.

One state legislator from an agricultural district was in the habit of bringing physical evidence to the statehouse in a vain effort to convince his urban colleagues of the vicious and destructive nature of the little red rascals—known to rural and urban legislators alike as "far'nts."

His standard exhibit was a gallon jug of disgruntled and irritable far'nts. He would challenge those who seemed not to take the threat seriously enough to "stick they hands in and see for themselves." To his continuing dismay, the blow-dried representatives of the new suburban South usually exhibited neither the guts to take him up on his challenge nor the wisdom to support the eradication program.

On the particular day in question, however, he brought to the House floor new evidence of far'nt atrocities, in the form of a rather pitiful-looking sweet potato. Standing in the well of the House as the vote on the appropriations measure was about to take place, he made one last appeal for understanding and sympathy from "my urbane colleagues.

"Before you vote," he pleaded, "I am going to pass this sweet potater out amongst you. I want you to see for yourselves what these awful critters can do.

"Look at that thing, my friends and fellow Georgians. It's been absolutely ridiculed by far'nts."

Ridiculed by far'nts.

Surely there is no better thought on which to end a book about the Carter White House and the press—nor a more appropriate benediction for me and all those with whom I worked in the White House—on both sides of the podium.

INDEX